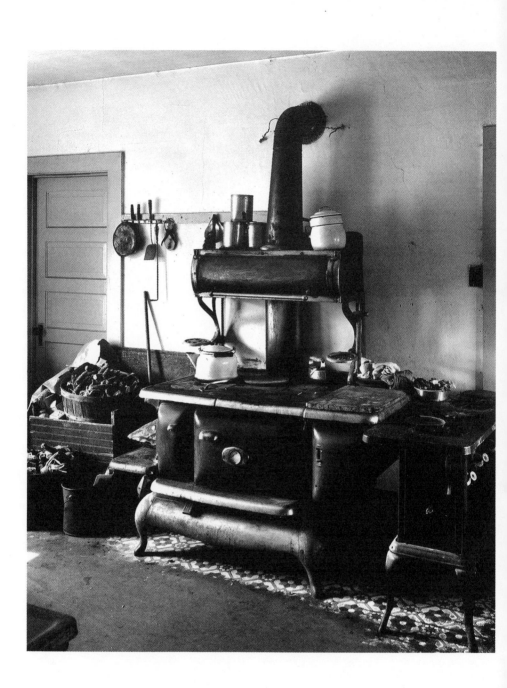

Our Sustainable Table

Edited by Robert Clark
for The Journal of Gastronomy

North Point Press   *San Francisco*   *1990*

This volume is the result of the kindness, labor,
and commitment of many people, and in particular of the writers who so willingly agreed to
contribute to it. The following individuals were
also indispensable in conceiving *Our Sustainable Table* and in seeing it through to publication: Alice Waters; Kirsten Bolin, Greg
Drescher, K. Dun Gifford, and Nancy Harmon
Jenkins; and Jennifer McDonald and Jack
Shoemaker of North Point Press.

LIBRARY OF CONGRESS
CATALOGING-IN-PUBLICATION DATA
Our sustainable table / edited by Robert Clark for the
American Institute of Wine & Food.
    p.   cm.
Originally published as the Journal of gastronomy,
v. 5, no. 2, summer/autumn 1989.
ISBN 0-86547-444-3.— ISBN 0-86547-445-1 (pbk.)
1. Agriculture — United States.   2. Diet — United
States.   3. Food.   I. Clark, Robert.   II. Ameri-
can Institute of Wine & Food.   III. Journal of
gastronomy.
S441.A483   1990
630'.973 — dc20   90-34729

North Point Press
850 Talbot Avenue
Berkeley, California
94706

Contents

Preface

Good farming means good food; anyone who cares about good food has a stake in good farming and in methods of food production, processing, and distribution that accord with the long-term health and sustainability of farmers, farming communities, and the land upon which they—and we—depend.

But discussions of food and food policy in America have been dominated for most of this century, and certainly since World War II, by questions of quantity rather than quality: "How much and at what price?" has often seemed more important than "how good and at what cost?" Our criteria for evaluating the ways in which we farm, market, shop, cook, and eat have largely been economic in nature, whereas how food relates to the land, our communities, and our public and private selves has been a question relegated to the margin of contemporary concerns. "The discipline proper to eating, of course, is not economics but agriculture," writes Wendell Berry. "The discipline proper to agriculture, which survives not just by production but by the return of wastes to the ground, is not economics but ecology." *Our Sustainable Table* is inspired by that remark. It shares Berry's distress with a society that divorces food production from food consumption while it shares his conviction that the fundamental element of our culture is agriculture: Since how we raise and eat our food reflects our husbandry of our selves, our communities, and the land that gives us life, we are what we eat not just in anthropological terms but also in moral and spiritual as well as economic and social terms.

Despite the apparent abundance that Americans enjoy, the

specter of scarcity in general and hunger in particular continues to shape our view of agriculture and food. Contemporary attitudes to both agriculture and eating are a response to the desire to produce the greatest quantity of food at the lowest price. To criticize the environmental or cultural effects of this is considered, at best, crankiness and elitism and, at worst, insensitivity to hunger itself. But for its critics, such a system merely substitutes for death by hunger the possibility of death by environmental degradation. Similarly, for those who care about how their food tastes and the ways in which preparing and sharing it resonate through their lives and communities, modern agricultural practice and the food it produces seem to have brought about plenty at the price of both private pleasure and the public good — food that fills the stomach but starves the soul.

In recent years, individuals and organizations throughout the world have been actively attempting to reestablish an agriculture that is consistent with environmental, human, and economic well-being: among the contributors to this book, Gary Nabhan's work to preserve native American food plants and crop diversity comes to mind, as do Wes Jackson's efforts to create an agriculture that complements rather than ignores the prairie ecosystem of our nation's breadbasket. At the same time, others have been working to restore food's aesthetic, psychological, social, and cultural dimension — to point out that food that tastes good and is good for you is not just a private indulgence but a force for sustaining families and communities, the end result of larger goods that benefit everyone: Alice Waters, for example, has created a restaurant many consider among the world's finest not just on the basis of carefully selected materials and good cooking but upon the idea that restaurants are a part of a web of interdependence that stretches from farm to market to cook. Frances Moore Lappé has been an influential force for an American diet that actively responds to the problems of global hunger and the economic and environmental crises of the Third World. These approaches suggest the possibility of nurturing a way of life that applies the same principles to individuals, communities, and their culture that sustainable agriculture brings to bear on farming.

Our Sustainable Table explores and encourages the link between the land and the table and urges the recovery of a vision of food in which agriculture and gastronomy are but two sides of the same coin. Lately, those concerned with growing food and those concerned with eating it have not had much to say to one another, tending to view the other side with suspicion or condescension. But the time is right to ask them to speak to one another's concerns: to ask those who think about farming to think about where food goes; and to ask those who think about cooking and eating to think about where food comes from—in short, to ask both sides to consider the manifold economic, social, and environmental import of how food is grown and the equally significant cultural, social, and psychological dimension of how it is eaten. The result, I hope, will be a sense of the thread that runs from a glass of wine or a simmering pot to family meals to markets to farms, and thence to the past traditions and future life of all our kind and of the earth itself.

Robert Clark
Editor

Our Sustainable Table

ONE

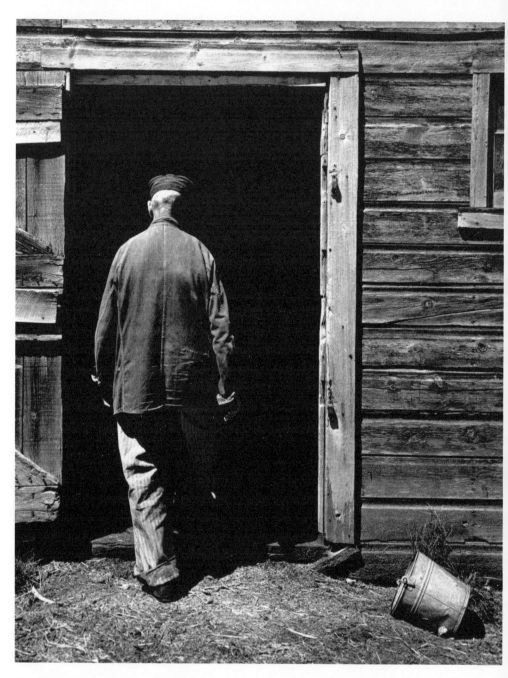

Uncle Harry, Home Place, Norfolk, Nebraska, 1947. Photo by Wright Morris.

Remember the Flowers
Paul Gruchow

My father was a farmer with no use for fashions. He married
and went into business for himself in the spring of 1946, raising
laying hens, vegetables, and berries on a seven-and-a-half-acre
truck farm. Small-scale horticulture was his real interest. For the
rest of his life, he devoted as much time and care to his gardens
and orchards and beehives as to his row crops. The eggs he sold
to the local candling plant, the berries and vegetables to the
local grocers. It was hard labor, mostly done with his hands and
a two-wheeled garden tractor, and it afforded a very meager
living. By 1947 he had infant twins as well as a wife to support,
and sometimes it took all the eggs in the henhouse just to buy
milk for the babies. In 1950, he rented 160 acres of land on
shares. The move required investing in a collection of ancient
farm machinery, but it also brought a barn and an above-ground
house with three rooms and electricity (the family had been
living in an unfinished basement). A decade later, my mother in-
herited 80 acres, giving our family the capital to finance the purchase of an additional 120 acres of land, about 40 acres of it in
pasture and meadow, so, in the last years of my father's life (he
died in 1970), he became a landholding farmer, although still on
a quite small scale.

The fifties and sixties were, of course, a time of great expansion in American agriculture, an expansion fueled by new

markets in war-ravaged Europe, by rising demand at home as the postwar baby boom took effect, and by the introduction in 1947 of 2,4-D, the first apparently safe and effective herbicide. 2,4-D was developed but never used as a chemical weapon during the war; it was to become, instead, a powerful tool in the industrialization of farming, a cheap alternative to the labor of cultivation. It had predictable consequences, although they were not predicted. One was the sudden obsolescence of many farmers; more than a million of them left the land in the fifties and crowded into cities, one of the great migrations in history. Another was overproduction; by the late fifties, the Soil Bank and the Ever-Normal granary had become part of the language of agriculture, the measuring wheel of the inspector from the Agricultural Stabilization and Conservation Service one of its tools, and ranks of Butler bins brimming with unmarketable grain among its architectural monuments. We had created a fantastic new food machine, like Strega Nona's pasta pot, but nobody knew how to turn it off.

That was the era in American agriculture when farming became not a vocation but a business, not a domestic art but a branch of industrial science—an era when the farm became not a legacy to be handed down from generation to generation but a capital asset from which one could reasonably expect an adequate return on investment, as measured in dollars and percents. What was the worth of a livelihood if it could not generate wealth?

It was also the era in which the American farm village disappeared. I lived in such a village in the fifties. It had a school and church, to which I walked. It had a social life, organized around the Christmas pageant, the end-of-school picnic, and the summer ice-cream social. We lived within sight and sound of neighbors who had children with whom we played.

One Sunday after dinner, as we called the noon meal, we children were summoned to a rare family conference. "We have something to tell you," my mother said, looking strangely radiant, "but it is a secret, and you are not to tell anyone. Do you understand?" Yes, my sister and I said, we understand, we will tell no one. "Remember, this is a secret," she said. Yes, yes, we said. "Well," she said, "your father and I want you to know that we are going to have a baby. When winter comes, you will have a new brother or sister. But this is a secret just between us for now. OK?" OK, we said, dancing with glee. We could hardly wait for Mother and Father to take their Sunday nap. (We had not yet discovered the connection between Sunday naps and new babies.) The instant they had settled down, we crept out the door, rushed to the next farm, and summoned the children.

"We have a secret," we said.

"Tell us! Tell us!"

What could we do, fiendishly pressed as we were? We told. "But don't tell anybody else," we said, absolving ourselves of responsibility.

By nightfall it was common knowledge in the neighborhood: "The Gruchows are expecting. Next winter."

In the sixties, the news probably would have remained a secret. We no longer lived in a neighborhood, in any practical sense. There was nobody we might have told; there were no other children within walking distance of our farm. There was no school; we rode the bus to town. The church was accessible only by car. Neighborhood social events had gone the way of the buggy. The gossip was of acquisitions, not of pregnancies. By the sixties, we lived, for the most part, alone. It was a triumph for productivity but not for humanity.

My father disregarded the new agriculture. He did not want land he could not care for. He refused to use the new chemicals. He was certain they were dangerous in ways that we would come eventually to understand. In any case, they took money, and all a hoe cost was some labor, of which he already had an adequate supply. At a time when a farmer's manhood was expressed in the size of his machines, he bought the smallest Fordson tractor available, a machine so insignificant that even I, a child, was embarrassed to drive it. When monoculture was the thing, he diversified. He expanded the sheep herd, started a business in goat's milk for families with infants allergic to cow's milk, planted potatoes and cucumbers, began a big apple orchard, trapped muskrats and mink in the winter. When the neighbors were razing the groves of empty farmsteads to make more land, he planted pines. When they tilled their meadows and plowed them, he dug a new pond in his for wild ducks.

It was not that he was indifferent to success. He studied the bulletins from the Agricultural Extension Service as assiduously as anybody. All winter, he pored over the reports of the crop variety trials, making notes of new hybrids to try. He kept his own careful performance records in the pocket notebooks handed out by the seed companies. He had a soil-testing kit and used it religiously. He meant to be the best farmer possible. It was just that he didn't see the connection between farming well and getting rich.

I had grown to adolescence and seen something of the world. He made me furious. One day I shouted at him, "You are like the soldier in the army who insists that everyone else is out of step!" I thought myself very clever.

He stared back at me, white with contempt. "Have you ever considered," he said, "the possibility that the soldier may be right?"

The reverse side of this, I suppose, is that my father was impractical. I dimly remember the search for a suitable piece of land when it became possible for him to buy one. He wanted two other farms much more than the one he actually bought. One had a single building on a treeless hillside, a European-style farmhouse, very long, in which everything was attached: House, barn, and henhouse all fell under a single roof, so that one could open a door and walk directly from the upstairs bedrooms into the haymow and from there down through a trapdoor into the animal quarters. We children were enthralled. There was an argument in the car on the way home.

"Think how efficient it would be," Father said.

"Absolutely not!" Mother said. "I will not live in a pigsty! You buy it, and you can go live there without me." It was clear that she meant it.

The other was a farm in the river bottom. The house on it was literally falling down. It was worse, unlikely as this was, than the house we were then living in. (Actually, I did not live in it myself, preferring a chicken coop that I shared one agonizing night with a skunk that had come in through a hole in the floor.) On the way home from our inspection visit, Father sounded childishly excited, the only time I ever saw him in such a state. Mother said nothing but halfway home she began to cry.

The first farm attracted my father because it included an enormous slough, the second because it was next to the river and consisted mainly of woodlands and rocky pastures. We were surrounded by farmers who thought that the most beautiful thing in the world was a flat field turned so thoroughly in the fall that nothing not perfectly black showed in it; who labored and conspired to turn every square inch of earth at their disposal to productive use; who tore out fences, cut down stray trees, drained marshes, plowed up farmyards and road ditches, forsook waterways in a desperate effort to wring the last dime out of a property; who saw any untilled acre as an offense against industriousness. But my father cherished the acres he couldn't farm as much as the ones he planted. He would no more have thought of buying a farm without some waste space in it than of moving to New York City and becoming a belly dancer.

We pulled into the yard at home after our trip to the farm along the river. He turned to Mother, who was staring sullenly out the window, and said, "I suppose you're right, honey. I suppose it really isn't practical." But you could tell that he said it out of resignation, not out of conviction.

Even now, when the fruits of farming as an industrial enterprise lie like so many rotting apples on the land, there are people who say that there is nothing wrong with agriculture that a better price for corn couldn't fix. They are right. If our success is to be measured in profit margins, let us guarantee the price of corn at ten dollars a bushel or a hundred dollars a bushel—it hardly matters what the figure is—and get on with our lives. The rich will grow very much richer, and the poor will still fail. Land prices will soar, and so will land abuse, and so will the prices suppliers charge. Rural population will continue to dwindle. The communities that survive will continue to struggle to maintain decently vigorous local institutions. Every issue of short-term justice and long-term sanity will remain. But those few who survive will become rich and powerful beyond their wildest dreams.

We in rural America have a long list of enemies: The government did it to us. The bankers did it to us. The grain cartels did it to us. The professors of agriculture did it to us. But the truth is, we did it to ourselves. We have had no agricultural policy that somebody in agriculture didn't press; and no lousy piece of advice ever came to ill unless somebody agreed to take it. The question every farmer has to answer, Wendell Berry once said, is this: "Would you rather have your neighbor's land or your neighbor?" We have made the choice over and over again, and, if we now have very few neighbors, we deserve to allocate some portion of the blame to ourselves.

There always was another choice. My father, for one, made it. It was his mark of excellence, the hilltop he made out of his life.

The heart of the matter is the question of economy. There are, essentially, only two ways to balance a checkbook. One is to make more, and the other is to make do with less. Of course, there are—it goes without saying—limits to the second strategy. Even Thoreau kept three chairs in his house at Walden Pond. "None is so poor that he need sit on a pumpkin," he explained, although I once lived in a house where we sat on empty sauerkraut kegs and am not aware that it did me or anyone else any harm.

My father lived in an industrial economy that he did not entirely spurn. He acquired property, occasionally purchased goods and services, participated in government farm programs, and received public support for his participation without, so far as I am aware, any tinge of regret. He believed in government and in its duty, not to mention its privilege, to manage our affairs (including his own) for the greatest good.

We had a serious falling out over this issue during the Vietnam War. I refused to fight, believing the war immoral; my father held passionately that I was wrong, that I might seek in every legal way to change the government's policy, but, so long as it was the policy, he said, I had a moral and a Christian obligation to do what it asked. During this time I gave a speech arguing otherwise. My father listened to it on the radio, and, when I went to the farm afterward to greet him, he met me at the front door and told me sadly that I was not welcome, that traitors were never welcome at his house. He was no isolationist, no believer in a world where it is every man for himself.

He did, nevertheless, practice a personal economy that was at considerable odds with the public economy. It was, for one thing, domestic. By this I mean that he, as a matter of principle, tried to do as much for himself as possible. In part, this meant being handy. He was not much of a consumer, but he spent a good deal of time at the local implement dealerships, studying the latest innovations and borrowing whatever ideas he found useful. He made an occasional visit to the blacksmith's shop for a bit of ironwork he wasn't equipped to handle, but otherwise he was self-sufficient. He was his own mechanic, his own carpenter, his own electrician, his own soil scientist, his own feed formulator, his own miller, his own veterinarian. Perhaps he died so young because he insisted, until it was too late, on being his own doctor. When he wanted something, he made it. If he couldn't make it, he did without or invented an alternative.

To some extent, my father's self-sufficiency was a matter of necessity, since he never had much money. But he seldom had much money mainly because he put so little value on it. I have little doubt that, had it been important to him, he could have made as much money as the next man. Self-sufficiency was also, for him, a matter of principle.

We raised our own food. It saved money, and he enjoyed it. But more than that, it seemed to him so logical, so obvious a thing to do that the rarity of it mystified him. That's what farmers do, he said: They raise food. If I am a farmer, he asked, and cannot even feed myself, what sort of farmer am I? Does a tailor hire somebody to make his own clothes? Does a cobbler send his shoes out to be fixed? So he raised livestock for meat and milk, kept bees for honey and chickens for eggs, maintained an orchard for fruit, tended vegetable and berry gardens, raised wheat and ground it himself into flour. He didn't have the imagination to do less.

I tried out on him once an idea I had picked up in a

vocational agriculture class. "Farming," I said to him, "is, after all, a business like any other. The purpose of farming is to make a living."

He flew into a rage. "Listen here, young man," he said. "The purpose of farming is to produce food for hungry people. It is a calling, not a living, and don't you ever forget it!"

In his economy, the guiding principle was the avoidance of waste. He understood the word to mean the unnecessary expenditure of life or the resources of life. Idling acres to curb excess production, therefore, made sense to him, but dumping milk didn't. Idle land was not wasted but merely lying fallow. It benefited the land, and, in any case, it was of some use to the rest of God's creation. But to spend resources to produce food and then to throw it out merely because you couldn't make a profit on it—that to him was waste, a kind of blasphemy. In the same way, it seemed to him not merely practical but morally good to heat our house with wood. It was, after all, available to us for the labor of harvesting it. Why should we burn coal, exhaustible and needing to be dug by somebody else, when we were perfectly capable of supplying our own replenishable heat at no expense to anyone? Shouldn't the coal be reserved for those who had no better alternative? My father's goal, in economic matters, as in the rest of life, was to be as little trouble to anybody else as possible.

I think he also meant to be as little trouble to himself as possible. He simplified his economic life so that the rest of his life might also be free and simple. In this he was Thoreauvian, although I doubt that he ever read Thoreau; and his habits, I think, gave his neighbors the same sort of trouble that Thoreau's gave *his* neighbors.

My father worked diligently at farming, but he refused to work at it slavishly. He rose at sunrise but never earlier and, at least in the summertime, frequently went to bed shortly after sundown. He believed in long, leisurely meals, napped religiously after lunch, and kept the Sabbath faithfully. Sometimes our neighbors, particularly during the planting and harvesting seasons, rose long before daylight and worked late into the night, the headlights of their machines piercing the midnight blackness. But when it got dark, the work on our farm stopped, no matter what the urgency of time or weather. I myself, as a teenager, rose at four-thirty in the morning in the summertime to work one job, took a break for lunch, and then frequently worked a second job until ten or ten-thirty in the evening. My father made no effort to stop me, but he made it perfectly clear that he regarded such effort as utter madness, as I myself do now.

He believed that a life of constant toil was badly led, a life God never intended for anyone. His farming was important to him: a noble and sacred calling. But other things were also important. He attended the flowering of wild plants, the singing of birds, the swarming of bees, the footprints of foxes. He cultivated his gardens. He walked in the woods. He prayed and meditated. In the winter, he helped his children to make igloos and snow tunnels. In the summer, he held them in his arms under the stars and sang cowboy songs to them in his sweet tenor voice.

For several years, we raised a couple of acres of cucumbers, an important cash crop. The project involved the entire family, and it might have been an unbearable drudgery. After the ground was plowed in the spring, everything was done by hand. The seeds were hand-planted in handmade hills, the patch was weeded with hoes, and, during the harvest season, we all spent three mornings a week, beginning before the dew had dried, picking the fruits, one by one, filling a peck basket, dumping it into the truck parked at the end of the field, filling another peck, and another, and another, until we were green and sticky to our elbows with the nauseating juice of cucumber vines and the sun was high in the sky and suffocatingly hot. It was back-breaking work, done on hands and knees, and excruciatingly boring, all the more because it had to be done meticulously. The cucumbers were graded by size, and the bigger they got, the less we were paid for them.

When we had gleaned the field, the cucumbers had to be hauled to the buying station in Willmar, forty miles away. We all piled into the truck, grateful for the chance simply to sit, and went together to Willmar, and, after we had sold the day's

harvest, we went to the lake there and swam away the late afternoon and had a picnic in the shade and drove home at dusk,
singing songs or falling happily asleep on our parents' shoulders.
In my father's economy, those half-days of lounging at the lake
were as vital as the mornings spent in the cucumber patch, and
without the one he would not have had the other.

Sometimes this attitude resulted in a casualness toward life
that could seem callous, although I think it was not. One fall
morning after we children had gone to school, the creosote in
the chimney of our house caught fire and started a blaze in the
attic. Father was miles away, on his parents' farm, plowing.
Mother was home alone. She ran to the neighbor's, borrowed
the telephone, called the fire department, and then called Grandmother and asked her to fetch Father from the fields. The fire
truck came, Grandmother came, several neighbors came, but not
my father.

He worked, as usual, until noon and then returned for lunch,
uncertain, of course, whether there was any lunch to be had. My
sister and I had also walked home from school for lunch and
were horrified when we rounded the grove, saw the commotion
of neighbors and fire fighters in the yard, and realized what had
happened. Father arrived after us. When Mother saw him, she
turned on him and yelled at him, the only time, I think, that she
defied him in public. "Where have you been!" she screamed.

"I have been plowing the eighty," he said calmly.

"While our house was burning!" she shouted.

"I know that," he said, "but there was nothing I could do to
stop it, was there? And I had work to do."

She was stunned into flaming silence.

He never did understand why she was so angry. As far as he
was concerned, you worried about what you could change, and
you accepted everything else. If a house burned, it was, after all,
only a house.

Thoreau went to Walden Pond, he said, to conduct an experiment. "I went to the woods because I wished to live deliberately,
to front only the essential facts of life, and see if I could not
learn what it had to teach, and not, when I came to die,

discover that I had not lived." He was quite explicit about the nature of his experiment. It was not, he said, a model for the ideal life, not an experiment he meant anybody else to copy. "I would not have any one adopt *my* mode of living on any account; for, beside that before he has fairly learned it I may have found out another for myself, I desire that there may be as many different persons in the world as possible; but I would have each one be very careful to find out and pursue *his own* way, and not his father's or his mother's or his neighbor's instead." And what his experiment taught him did not, in fact, have anything to do with living "cheaply or meanly." The lesson was in values, not in prices. "I learned this, at least, by my experiment: that if one advances confidently in the direction of his dreams, and endeavors to live the life which he has imagined, he will meet with a success unexpected in common hours. He will put some things behind, will pass an invisible boundary; new, universal, and more liberal laws will begin to establish themselves around and within him; or the old laws be expanded, and interpreted in his favor in a more liberal sense, and he will live with the license of a higher order of beings. In proportion as he simplifies his life, the laws of the universe will appear less complex, and solitude will not be solitude, nor poverty poverty, nor weakness weakness. . . . Superfluous wealth can buy superfluities only. Money is not required to buy one necessary of the soul."

Thoreau's experiment has raised a nervous defensiveness in a long line of critics, beginning with Thoreau's own best friend, Emerson, who admired him and helped to establish his reputation, but who also dismissed him at his funeral, in a memorable phrase, as "the captain of a huckleberry party."

We have a public conception of moral responsibility. Despite the long thread of individualism running through our culture, we tend to believe that whatever is good is good in the collective sense. We may admire Thoreau and his descendants, Gandhi and Martin Luther King Jr., for the high-mindedness of their sentiments, but we are at the same time suspicious of a philosophy that seems so personal, so intensely directed at the individual life. To seek by public means to change the evil in our lives—

that we can honor and respect. But simply to refuse, as one human being, acting alone, to participate in evil—that seems to us somehow dangerous, selfish, too piddling to make much practical difference. How could Thoreau, we want to know, busy himself, in good conscience, as the "self-appointed inspector of snowstorms" when the much greater turbulence of slavery was raging all around? It is true that he championed John Brown, spoke passionately in Concord and elsewhere in favor of abolition, and perhaps assisted a traveler or two on the Underground Railroad to freedom in Canada, but it is also true that Thoreau was no reformer. His heart wasn't in it. He would sooner have gone walking in the woods. How dare such a man pretend to any moral superiority?

There are two classes of moralists: those who seek to improve the quality of other people's lives, and those who are content to improve their own lives. There are professors of morality, and there are practitioners of it; the categories tend to be exclusive. Nothing is so terrifying as a demonstration of principle. Emerson preached Nature; Thoreau embraced nature; it is Thoreau, of course, who ultimately strikes us as dangerous. It is one thing to decry the rat race, to utter ringing declarations against it, to write clever stories exposing its follies—that is the good and honorable work of moralists. It is quite another thing to quit the rat race, to drop out, to refuse to run any further— that is the work of the individualist. It is offensive because it is impolite; it makes the rebuke personal; the individualist calls not his or her behavior into question, but mine. The moralist believes in the necessity of enemies, the individualist in their irrelevance.

It was so with my father. He went to the same church as his neighbors, confessed the same creed, partook of the same absolution. He heard the same preaching: "Take no thought for the morrow," and "Lay not up treasures on earth, where moth and rust doth corrupt," and "It is harder for a rich man to enter into heaven than for a camel to pass through the eye of a needle." But he made people nervous because he not only professed these beliefs, he practiced them. When he heard that his house was burning, he went on with the plowing. People said of him what is always said of such people: How selfish, how impractical, what a shame for his family! Think what he might have done if he had ever tried to make something of himself!

One spring night my father went to bed, fell asleep, and never awoke. He died as quietly, as uncomplainingly, as he had lived. It was an awkward moment for a farmer to die, too late in the season to secure someone else to run the land. He had thought of that. In the papers he left behind was a set of instructions for Mother: diagrams of the farm, notes on what to plant where and when, instructions on the management and harvesting of the crops, on the proper care of the machinery, on the arcane details of the year's farm program—everything Mother needed to know to operate the farm herself that summer, as she did, triumphantly.

Among the instructions he left behind was a plan for the flower beds in the yard, complete with planting charts, species names, and notes about when each variety would bloom and what color it would be. Even in death the flowers mattered to him. They were a reminder, which I have sometimes betrayed but never forgotten, of all that is genuinely important in life.

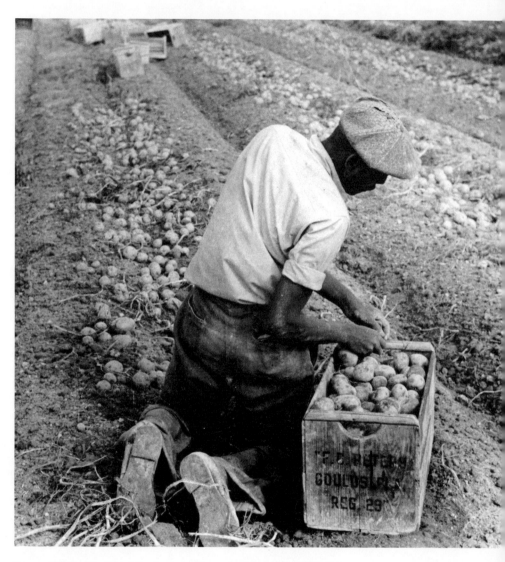

Potato Picker, Florida, March 1939. Photo by Mary Post Wolcott.

The Gleaners
Will Weaver

That first season the gleaners came out only at sundown. They parked their vehicles, battered Chevrolets and rusted Datsun pickups, well away from each other on the road that ran by the field. Caps pulled low on their foreheads, gunnysack shawls across their backs, the gleaners crossed the ditch and entered the field. Under a pink and blue sky, the air belled with September chill, the gleaners had eyes only for the ground, for the black, heaved furrows, the damp and tangled vines at their feet. They had come to look for potatoes that the mechanical harvester had missed or discarded.

There—a fat, muddy russet, big as a man's hand.

There—in the trough of the irrigator's wheel, another fat one.

There—in a clump of vines, two smaller potatoes.

Ahead—beside a heavy stone brightly scarred, among a small maze of bootprints and a blacker stain of oil, a whole scattering of potatoes.

Stoop, stoop, and stoop again: In this way the gleaners moved down the field. Their progress was measured against the dark silhouette of the irrigator, its long drooping lengths of pipes and tall stilt legs. Intermittently, like prairie dogs rising for a quick look, the gleaners stood fully erect to measure their distance from the other pickers and from the road and their own cars. Then they quickly bent again to their work. In the fading light, humps grew on the gleaners' backs as the weight of potatoes stooped their shapes ever lower until, in the purple dark, they staggered back to their cars. Sacks thudded. Trunk lids slammed. Engines raced and gravel chattered sharply against wheel wells as their vehicles accelerated away without headlights toward the highway.

The second season the gleaners came out earlier in the evening. Some appeared already in the afternoon, and the boldest waited in their cars beside the potato fields as harvesters worked the last rows. Word was that Universal Potato Company didn't care. It had bigger things to worry about, things like hot spots in one of the storage bins, nailing down the Burger King contract, the union sniffing around. Universal Potato wasn't about to bother people who picked up a few stray spuds. Just don't drive in the fields or otherwise pack down the dirt—that was the unofficial word. Otherwise, have at them. Plenty of spuds for the taking. Enough for the whole town of Flatwater (population 2,650)—that was the word in the cafés and stores on Main Street. With spuds free for the picking, why would a person even fool with potatoes at home in the garden?

That second autumn other types of vehicles began to drive slowly along the potato fields. These were newer, shinier cars: Ford sedans, late-model Pontiacs, an occasional older Cadillac. Often they stopped, amber parking lights on, radios playing faintly through open windows as the cars' occupants watched the gleaners. The spectators were mostly older retired couples, people like Shirley Anderson and her husband, John.

"Look at them," Shirley remarked, staring past her husband at the gleaners. "Don't it remind you of the depression?" She was seventy-four, had short white curly hair, and wore a gauzy blue head scarf set loosely over her permanent and knotted tightly at the chin. She was neatly dressed in knit pants, blouse, and sweater. Out of the side of her eyes she watched for her husband's reaction.

John's heavy white eyebrows drooped slightly as he squinted. He remained silent, hands wrapped around the steering wheel.

"You wouldn't think, in modern times like these, a person would ever see this, would you?" Shirley said, clucking her tongue briefly. She watched as a heavyset woman stooped for a potato, then another and another like a fat old hen picking her way across a chicken yard. She plucked six spuds in quick succession. Shirley felt her heart pick up a beat.

"Depression days are coming again," John said. He clenched the steering wheel and his fingers reddened. "Things can't go on the way they are!"

"Some people would agree with you," Shirley said quickly. She didn't want to anger him, have him drive off. It had been difficult enough getting him to take her on the dirt roads past the potato fields. Their car was a white 1976 Oldsmobile with 24,532 miles on the odometer and no rust spots or paint chips — a town car. Shirley did not drive. She had never had a license.

"I mean, why can't people raise their own food, like we do?" She turned the angle of her vision an inch so as to watch him more closely.

He continued to stare out into the field somewhere.

Shirley turned her eyes back to the gleaners. The fat woman dragged her gunnysack forward. Shirley's heart beat slightly faster still, and she reached underneath her sweater to touch the plastic bag that she had brought along.

"Easier to steal them, everybody steals nowadays," John said. His voice rose sharply.

Shirley swung her gaze away, out her side window and across the road to a drifting hawk that she pretended had caught her interest. With John she had to go carefully. At age seventy-nine he was an increasingly silent, unpredictable man. Conversation with him was like speaking with their son who lived in Alaska. His phone was hooked up to a satellite, and the words had to bounce off something (was it the earth or was it the satellite? she could never remember), then float back. There was a delay. You had to wait. You couldn't talk fast and you couldn't interrupt.

"Though," Shirley said evenly, looking back to the potato field, "you couldn't really call it stealing, could you?" She paused. "I mean, Universal would just plow them under, wouldn't they?"

John stared across the field. Shirley watched the fat woman shake a clump of potato vines. Dirt showered in the sunlight.

"Their potatoes are poison," John said. "The chemicals!"

Shirley waited. She watched the big woman stoop five more times, then drag her bag forward, leaning into the task, using both hands now.

"Oh, I don't know about that," Shirley said, drawing in a little whistle of air through her teeth to show that she wasn't in a hurry or in any way serious about the topic at hand. "Some people say they taste just as good as homegrown." Inside her sweater, she gathered up the plastic bag.

A car came toward them from behind. Shirley turned quickly to look at the battered pickup that rattled past, its dust rolling briefly upward, then tilting slowly toward the ditch. John, staring into the sunset, did not even turn his head.

She eyed her husband for a long moment, then said, "Maybe we should give them a try." She laughed briefly—loud enough so that he was certain to hear. "Why don't I just step out there and find us a couple of spuds for our supper?"

In the silence a small airplane droned overhead. Its single red light blinked slowly across the sky, crawling toward the Dakotas. Suddenly John's hand dropped from the wheel onto the gearshift and the car lurched forward.

They passed a second potato field where a shiny blue car parked in the shallow ditch drew Shirley's eyes. A car from town. A familiar car, though she couldn't put the person's name to it. The owner, a well-dressed woman about her own age, with white hair and pink scarf tied at the chin, was a few yards behind in the field. She carried a white plastic grocery bag that could only come from Marketplace Food and Deli, the new grocery store in town. Shirley leaned forward through her window to squint at the woman who, at the same moment, looked toward the road. It was Thelma Haynes, a widow who worked in the floral shop at Marketplace Food and Deli. Their eyes locked. Thelma turned quickly away toward the field; Shirley ducked her head out of sight below the car's window.

John turned to stare at her. Shirley pretended to see something on the floor, then sat up straight again. The car moved on. As they drove she kept her eyes peeled, as usual, for cars over the center, for farm implements or stray animals on the road, but her mind was filled with another vision: Thelma Haynes's plastic grocery bag. It was blooming white on top, hanging dark and heavy below. Slowly Shirley's gaze swung around to the interior of the Oldsmobile. She began to stare at the steering wheel. The dashboard. The levers. She watched the pedals. How he positioned his feet. She knew which pedal stopped the car, which gave it gas. The brake. The gas pedal. Two pedals, two feet. She looked at the shift lever. The little window above the steering wheel said, "P R D 2 1." Momentarily she thought of the "Wheel of Fortune" game show. How most people chose the letters "R S T L E." How she often figured out the phrase long before the contestants. How most things could be figured out if a person paid attention. She looked back to her husband's hands, where he positioned them on the steering wheel.

Later, as they drove on blacktop, a heavy, deep-fat smell drew her gaze to the Universal Potato Company, a long, airport-hangar-sized building that stood at the edge of town. Its walls were concrete, windowless panels, and high atop the gray front was the company's symbol, a giant potato, which radiated yellow-painted sunbeams from its brown body. Above the potato, steam billowed from vents and shiny turbines that spun out a hot, starchy smell of french fries. It was the odor of progress — the aroma of jobs.

Universal Potato had come to northwestern Minnesota from Idaho where the land was tired and the water expensive. Around Flatwater, the land, graded perfectly flat by some long-ago glacier, was fresh, sandy loam on top with clean gravel below and a water table that rose up to within twenty feet of daylight. The combination was ideal for irrigation and big machinery. It was a wonder, Shirley thought, that farmers around here had not thought of growing potatoes themselves.

But people, especially farmers, were creatures of habit. Before potatoes this land had supported only dairy cows, and barely enough of them for farmers to scratch out a living. Shirley had grown up on such a farm — the white house, the red sheds, the black hills of manure that rose up in winter behind the barn. In spring the manure went back onto the fields and the whole country stank so strongly that, while waiting for the school bus, her eyes had always run tears; if she tied her head scarf across her face to cover her nose, bandit style, then her hair had smelled of manure when she arrived at school. There were kids, rough-looking boys and tomboy girls, who had always smelled of the barn because they did chores before school, and she had steered clear of them. Her friends were town kids.

After high school Shirley took a teller's position at First Farmer's Bank and married John Anderson, who ran the hardware store. Her bank was the most modern building in town with its fluorescent lights and a continual, cool, humming breath of air-conditioning. In town the only time she had to smell manure was when farmers came in for their loans.

Looking back, something Shirley did often after she retired, she saw a trend among the farmers who came to the bank. It had to do with the smell of manure. In the 1950s only a few farmers came in for loans, and they stank strongly of cow dung and occasionally of DDT. In the 1960s more farmers came for loans. They smelled sweeter and dustier with the scent of commercial fertilizers such as nitrogen, phosphate, and sulfur, along with the orange-rind aroma of 2,4-D, the brush and slough-grass killer. In the 1970s, when First Farmer's grew in assets from $1 million to $6 million, the farmers had come in droves. More chairs were added to the waiting room, and their fabric soon gave off the sharper, nose-itching smell of agrichemicals: herbicides; pesticides; Atrazine, Roundup, Lorsban. By the end of the 1970s the odor of manure was gone altogether. Farmers dressed better, sometimes even wearing ties for their meetings with the loan officers. By 1980, when First Farmer's built its new building and simplified its name to First Bank, the farmers had at long last joined modern times. And Shirley, as retired chief teller, was proud to have played a part.

Of course, with changing times some things were lost. The twenty-cow dairy farm had pretty well disappeared by 1975, and even forty cows were hardly enough nowadays. But an omelet could not be made without first breaking the eggs; survival of the fittest, that was the way Shirley saw it. The farmers who could adapt changed to irrigation. Square fields turned round under the slowly circling irrigators that sprinkled corn day and night through July and August. Dairy barns, empty of cows, their stanchions removed, now leaked number-two yellow corn from their windowsills and ventilators. Farmers read market news, went to seminars in Minneapolis or Fargo, stayed in touch with world events.

Those who didn't lost out, went under. In the bank Shirley had seen it close-up. If it was sad initially—the dispersal auctions in particular—a farmer losing his land wasn't as bad as people had made it out to be, for then the potato growers had arrived. Universal Potato Company gave top prices for irrigable land and usually gave the farmers jobs besides. Farmers stayed on in their own homes, continued to work their own land. Now they drove tractors and harvesters that belonged to Universal Potato, and they no longer had to worry about maintenance, about breakdowns, about the high price of parts. In the evening there were no barn chores, no more getting up at midnight to birth a calf. For the first time in their lives, the men had time to watch TV, to go fishing on occasion or drive their families on a Saturday afternoon over to the mall in Fargo.

In Flatwater the stores improved. A Hardee's came to town, and Marketplace Food and Deli followed. An antique store opened on Main Street where old milk cans and separators were the best sellers. Sometimes Shirley browsed through the store, clucking her tongue at the things people would buy. A pedal grindstone. Blue mason jars. Wooden kraut cutters. Washboards. She wondered what had become of things like her family's old ice chest, the crank phone; some items were worth an astounding amount of money. But antiques were a laugh. Shirley had grown up with antiques. Why would she want to buy them back? She had no desire to return to the old days. To depression days. To the flat frozen fields, the black winter mountains of manure.

The next morning, early, Shirley woke up with a vision of white. Frost. She sat up in bed, remembering she had not covered the squash or the muskmelons. Quickly she dressed, put on a jacket and rubber boots, and went out. A white rime of frost coated the steps, and beyond it—she saw immediately—the tall squash plants lay flattened and brown in the garden. On their shrunken vines the cantaloupes sat up high and shiny like skulls. She muttered under her breath.

In the wet, flattened garden, the only green was a row of peas and carrots that John had planted. Somehow, in planting, he had gotten the seeds into the same trench. In June the row had come up frothy green like a wave of seawater rising from the garden, threatening to spill over everything. By late July the row had crested, collapsed under its own weight, and delivered no peas and no carrots. It remained now in September so dense and junglelike that even frost could not penetrate it.

No matter. The garden was finished now, and good riddance, Shirley thought. She looked briefly back to the house, then around at the neighborhood. The houses nearby were narrow, white, and tall with dark, steep-pitched roofs and caragana and lilac bushes rising up untrimmed toward the windows where shades remained pulled; their neighbors, all older couples like themselves, were still sleeping. They weren't worrying about gardens and frost. All of them had long ago figured out that it was cheaper to buy food. John and Shirley had the only garden. Once she had drawn up a list of garden expenses for John. It had sent him into a rage, and she had not spoken of it again.

Now she walked along the mess of pea vines and carrots to the four rows of potatoes where there was a plant here, a plant there. Long gaps of weedy dirt between. Had he planted them too deeply? Cut the seed potatoes wrong, left them with no eye? Put the eye staring down, sent its white shoot on a death march to China? It didn't matter now.

Shirley went to get the wheelbarrow for the squash and melons. In the garage she paused by the Oldsmobile. In the dim light from the window, the car's paint glowed whitely. She ran a finger along its roof, then down the cool window glass to the chrome door handle. Quietly opening the door, she eased into the driver's seat. Her heartbeat immediately picked up speed. She raised her hands to the steering wheel. The little grooves — how well they fit the fingers! She turned the wheel left and right. She sat there staring through the windshield and the garage window, beyond which she could see only sky and the vague, darker peaks of the neighbors' roofs. She sat there until she heard shouting in the garden.

She blinked.

"They're stealing!" John was shouting.

Shirley scrambled from the car and found John in the garden in his pajamas, with no jacket, no shoes, shouting.

"The kids, they're stealing again!" He waved his arms.

"Here! Hush!" Shirley called. "Stop that crazy talk!"

"The kids," John said. "Look at the garden. It's all gone."

"There's no stealing because there's nothing to steal," Shirley said. She grabbed his arms, and her words came out faster than she wanted, but she couldn't slow them or pull them back. "That stealing stuff is all in your mind because your mind is not so good anymore—you can see that by the way things are planted."

John let his eyes fall slowly to the thick green row of peas and carrots.

"You're too old to plant a garden, just like I'm too old to work in one," Shirley said. "Things change and you've got to get that into your head. Don't you see," she said, softer now, "we're old. Old."

In a long, slow turning of his head, John brought his gaze around to hers. The morning light shone in his eyes, and for an instant she saw him as he had been when he was a young man. Then he looked down, down to his own hands. He stared at his fingers, his palms, turned them over, then back, then over again.

She went to him. "Come on in," she said.

He let himself be led into the house.

Later in the morning, since it was Saturday, they went grocery shopping as usual. John drove. Shirley watched him warily, but he drove well enough, and they arrived at Marketplace Food and Deli without trouble.

"You want to come in this time?" Shirley said.

John looked across the parking lot to the new store. Marketplace had slanting copper-colored angles to its metal roof and several colored flags flying on top; it was what Shirley imagined a Spanish train station must look like. There was also a drive-up window for grocery pickup that kept people out of the rain and snow and sun. And under one roof, it offered a bakery, coffee shop, florist's shop, video section, and film-processing station, as well as the deli and grocery aisles that went on and on under bright fluorescent lights.

"Too big," John said. "A person could get lost in there."

"Well, sit there then," she said with some relief. "I'll be right back. You got that?"

Halfway across the parking lot, she looked back to see him, alone in the car, nodding yes.

Inside the store, from the smell of the bakery Shirley realized she had not finished her own breakfast. Now she had to shop on an empty stomach, something she tried never to do; it always ran up the grocery bill. She found a cart and, before moving an inch, made herself read aloud the list. "Crisco. Yeast. Baking soda. Flour. Milk. Turkey (leg). Navy beans. Hand soap."

In produce she passed by eggplants, jalapeño peppers, kiwifruit, artichokes, gingerroot, guavas—who in this town ate such things? Briefly she hefted an avocado, then put it back. At home she had jars and jars of perfectly good green beans and tomatoes and pickled carrots. She found Idaho red potatoes, a ten-pound plastic bag for $3.99! She hefted the bag, held it up toward the light. The potatoes were all as firm and round as apples and scrubbed a fresh, chapped red. She thought of the scattering of her own potatoes—droopy, sprouted, and brown—that remained in the root cellar. She let the bag of Idaho potatoes balance on the edge of her cart. She turned it sideways for another look. Finally she thudded the sack back onto its shelf.

In fruits she passed baby coconuts, Asian pears, papayas, and other odd-duck items until she reached California seedless grapes. Still sixty-nine cents a pound, though down a nickel since last Saturday. She moved on. Blue plums caught her eye, and she stopped to smell them, squeeze their little purple bellies. Her own stomach growled. She swallowed, checked her list, then tore off a plastic bag and chose two of the fattest plums.

The turkey leg took longer. "Most people want the breasts," the manager said cheerfully. He was a round-faced man who wore a white plastic hat with a short bill; as he dug through the freezer bin, the round white packages clacked against each other. "I'll have to look in back," he said.

As she waited, she added up the total so far, then thought about eating one of the plums. But it would not be washed, and, besides, someone might think she was not going to pay for it.

The manager appeared in the doorway. "Fresh or frozen?"

"Frozen," Shirley said quickly.

Heading toward hand soap, she passed through the feminine-products section, shelf after shelf of shields, liners, rinses, all packaged with drawings of women in white dresses in a sunny field of daisies or at the seashore where their long hair blew lightly in a breeze. She thought of her own cotton that she had washed every month, of it hanging on the far end of the clothesline, waving in the wind during the summer, swinging stiffly in winter. Today there was none of that for her. As she passed by the little plastic boxes and packets, she had to look twice to figure out what some of the things were for.

In the soap section she sneezed twice—had to steady herself against her cart until the dizziness passed. Coming down the final aisle, Shirley was so hungry that she held tightly to the cart and let it pull her along. Rounding the corner, she smelled flowers and at the same moment saw Thelma Haynes. Thelma was dressed in a white apron with a fresh carnation on her blouse, her hair done up far too blue; she stood polishing the glass counter of the floral shop.

"Shirley Anderson," Thelma called out in an artificially cheery voice, "what can I do for you today?"

"Me? Oh, no, just the groceries," Shirley said.

"Special on fresh carnations," Thelma said brightly.

"I grow my own flowers," Shirley said immediately. The fool idea that she didn't drove away her hunger.

"Well, they are cheaper that way," Thelma said, lowering her voice. A young manager-type fellow passed. He wore a short-sleeved white shirt and a thin black tie, and Thelma turned quickly to adjust some dried flowers in a fancy teakettle pot.

"Everything is too high-priced," Shirley said.

Thelma fussed with the stems. Weeds really. Spray-painted weeds.

"Take potatoes," Shirley said, narrowing her eyes slightly.

"Nearly forty cents a pound."

For a moment Thelma was silent. Her small blue eyes flickered briefly around her before they came back to Shirley. "I guess it depends on where you get them," Thelma said.

"Yes. I suppose it does," Shirley said.

"You know how many potatoes I've got?" Thelma whispered. Her eyes widened momentarily, a sudden surge of light.

Shirley held tighter to the cart's handle.

"Twelve bushel. Maybe fifteen. They take up the whole closet and part of the bedroom of my apartment," Thelma said. She giggled briefly.

Shirley felt the grocery cart push her backward an inch.

Thelma leaned forward across her counter. "I tell myself I won't go out there again," she whispered, "but the next thing I know, there I am."

"You could give some away!"

Thelma narrowed her eyes.

"Other people, who can't get around by themselves, they might like some of those potatoes," Shirley said. She leaned slightly forward.

Thelma turned sideways to wipe at something on the glass, then gave Shirley a sidelong look. "I don't know. I've got myself to think of."

"Fifteen bushel!" Shirley said.

Thelma blinked and for a moment her eyes widened again as they took in the store behind—the aisles, the displays, the people with their carts, the children. "No one knows what's going to happen," she whispered. "You could live on potatoes if you had to."

At the till Shirley waited behind a heavyset woman with a cart topped off with two twelve-packs of Mountain Dew. She breathed lightly through her mouth as she watched the cashier swing the items across the red light that burned beneath the counter. The beeping went on and on. To speed things up when her turn came, Shirley counted out exact change: $13.68. She clutched the money. Her hand shook slightly. Ahead, as the beeping of the groceries went on, the fat woman stood leafing through a *Teen Beat* magazine; she had no idea of what things cost, Shirley realized. What kind of person did not know the price of things? She felt a fine cool sweat begin to come on her forehead.

When Shirley at last passed through the electric doors, the grocery boy behind her, the wide parking lot outside tilted for an instant—then righted itself—then tilted again.

"Lady, are you all right?" the boy said. His voice sounded faraway.

"Of course I'm all right," Shirley said. "Just a little hungry."

For some reason he grabbed her, roughly, and the next thing she saw was his face staring down at her. She was lying on the asphalt.

"Call 911!" the boy was shouting.

"No!" Shirley said sharply. The cost of an ambulance gave her a surge of energy, and she sat up. "Those are my groceries," she said quickly to the boy. Her sack lay tipped over on the asphalt. She struggled to her feet and shook her finger at him. "I paid good money for those!"

At twilight, in the chilly, silent yard, Shirley stood beside their bedroom window and listened. She had slept all afternoon, and now it was John who snored on. He was out for the night. And so was she.

Wearing one of his old caps and carrying a flat flour sack over her shoulder, Shirley went to the garage. There she stowed the bag in the trunk of the Oldsmobile, then got behind the wheel. Taking a deep breath, she started the engine.

Its noise made her flinch and duck her head for a moment. Then she looked up, swallowed, and began to back out of the garage. On the street she paused to catch her breath, then put the little arrow on "D" and got ready. She wrapped her fingers tightly around the wheel, her fingernails biting back into her palms, and felt her heart beating around and around the wide, hard hoop of the wheel. Or maybe it was the humming pulse of the engine she felt. Swallowing once more, she took her foot off the brake.

She crossed Main Street without event. On the side streets,

each time a car approached she held her breath and, at the last moment as they passed, jammed shut her eyes. Remarkably, when she opened them, the street was clear again.

As she headed toward the city limits, two cars flashed their lights at her. Then a third. Was she too far over? What was she doing wrong? Cars passed her from both directions, sometimes tooting, sometimes flashing their lights. The headlights! She began to pull buttons along the dashboard—the wipers came on—until yellow beams shot down the road in front of her. After that she set her jaw and brought the Cutlass up to forty.

In a few minutes she began to look for the dirt road that turned west toward the potato fields. In gray dusk everything was smaller, narrower, farther off, a flat dusky plate with an occasional looming grove of trees, and she almost missed the road. Turning sharply, the car tilted over the corner, bounced once on something—a stone—that clinked underneath, then found the gravel road again. She drove another mile, then another and another. About to turn back, she saw, in silhouette, stretched across the field, the long black spine of an irrigator.

A car was just pulling away from the field. Shirley sped up suddenly, then braked to a halt with a final lurch. From the bottom of her sack she lifted the cool heavy cylinder of the flashlight, checked its beam, then headed quickly down and across the ditch. She had not walked twenty steps before the narrow beam of her light speared a potato.

Then another.

And another.

Rapidly she dropped them into the sack.

But they were so small. In the next moment she realized that these were potatoes other people had passed by. She dumped them from her sack and headed deeper into the field. Ten minutes later she found a furrow that no footprints had followed, and there she began to find real potatoes. Heavy-bodied russets. One would make a meal. She began to think of them that way. Meal.

Meal.

Meal.

Meal.

She hurried forward, following her light, stooping and stooping again, the sack bouncing on her back. In what seemed no time, the neck of the sack began to chafe sharply across her shoulder, and her arm was cramping.

She stopped. She looked back toward the road where the Oldsmobile, small and far away, drew light from the falling dark and glowed like a lighthouse beacon. She pressed on. Three more, she told herself—three more *good* ones. One by one she found them—five, actually—then made herself turn back.

By the time she reached the Oldsmobile, her breath came in short gasps. Her arms were numb. She slumped against the car and tried to breathe evenly. It took her several minutes to regain her strength, and as she stared off across the dark she gradually came to see how few lights there were on the land. A white pinprick of a yard lamp here and there. Four, possibly five farms if she looked in all directions. That was all.

She began to think of neighbors from her childhood. The van den Eykels. The Lanes. The Grunheims. The Niskanens. The Petersons. She wondered what had become of them. Other memories, images from childhood, rose up from the darkness. The bright Surge milking kettle that her father had swung from cow to cow. The oiled leather surcingle strap from which the milker had hung like a second belly beneath the cow. The Watkin's salesman with the glass eye and the sweet jars of orange and purple nectar that her mother had bought from him. The slivers of ice her father had chipped from the blocks that he fished, with black tongs, from beneath wet sawdust. The April melting, the wide field ponds where she and the other farm kids had sailed shingle boats with corn-shuck sails. Where had it all gone?

She had grown up, of course, and things had changed, as they must. Still leaning against the trunk, she looked back toward Flatwater. Her town glowed under a fuzzy cap of orange. Those new sodium-vapor streetlights. The town did not need to be lit up so brightly, she suddenly thought, and certainly not all night. One needed just enough light to see by. She switched on her flashlight again and turned its beam far out into the night. Where its light stopped, she imagined, was where the present ended and the past began. She thought about that for a moment. Abruptly she swung the light back into the trunk. Its yellow glow bobbed in steady rhythm as she began to count potatoes. Afterward, she shouldered the empty sack and turned the light, once again, onto the dark field.

A Sense of Place

Edward Behr

Back in the 1960s, nearly everyone who lived in the northeastern
corner of Vermont was born here. I moved to this region in
1973, part of the first wave of outsiders to arrive. At that time
there were a number of abandoned houses, and rents and land
were cheap. It didn't seem surprising. In this cold part of the
world the trees are bare of leaves during most of the year. Spring
is sudden and quick, and summer is short. In a bad year the
frosts are only sixty days apart, though there is warm weather
before and after. Those of us who came from elsewhere stayed
in spite of the cold because this place was beautiful, inexpensive,
and rural.

The three northeasternmost counties of Vermont are called
the Northeast Kingdom. In some parts, farms dominate the
landscape, but in many areas there remains as much wilderness as human presence. Few buildings appear in the distant
views of hills and forests. Each summer more of the fields that
make the landscape picturesque revert to woods, even as more
houses are built.

So much nature can create a pathos about the small scale of
human construction. Old houses, new ranch houses, even the
few commercial downtowns look frail when they are set against
hills and mountains. In summer, green foliage closes in some of
the distant views and the scale is more intimate. And in areas
where new ranch houses and commercial development have
become the norm, the contrast between buildings and the grand
scheme of nature begins to disappear. Indeed, the emptiness is
filling up.

I don't like to think about this. I don't read the local

newspapers because I find the changes painful. I prefer the illusion that my surroundings are timeless, permanent. But last fall I was talking to our county agricultural extension agent, Dennis Kauppila, when I blundered onto the subject of farm income. Dennis arrived in Vermont at about the same time I did. He grew up in Detroit, and his Finnish last name stands out among the mostly English, Scottish, Swedish, and French-Canadian names around here. He worked at odd jobs, generally as a farmhand, for seven years until he went to the state university to finish his bachelor's degree and get a master's in agricultural economics. Almost 90 percent of northern New England farms are dairy farms, and it is now my friend's job to do what he can to help them. He probably sees a disproportionate number of farmers who are in rough shape. For him, farm income—or lack of it—is an emotional subject.

Dennis was quick to offer figures for average income in several northeastern states: Last year, farms with jersey or guernsey cows had a cash income of $11,568, and farms with heavy milkers like holsteins had a cash income of $16,887. Many families actually live on this income, buying food and clothing, raising children, and paying for all other expenses, with little to spare for nonessentials.

A few years ago this news wouldn't have taken me by surprise, but now it did. Northeastern farmers have always struggled, but today farms that were worth $25,000 only twenty years ago are changing hands for $200,000 and more, and certainly conventional city and suburban housing costs are higher than that. I had simply failed to think that nothing had occurred to raise farm income. It isn't hard to see that the disparity between the value of the farmer's labor and the value of his land bodes ill for many farms in the populous East. (Already on marginal farms the farmer sometimes works at another part-time job to support the farm.) The price of milk is determined by more inexpensively produced milk from western farms. In the East, farmers sell out at a slow but steady rate; their land is developed, or in some areas the fields return to woods. After I learned the dispiriting figures on income, my thoughts began to turn to the subject I would rather avoid: the transformation of the deep countryside of the northeast—the places that feel profoundly rural.

People I know who don't live in the country assume that the country, the real country, is still out there. Perhaps, visiting it so seldom, they wouldn't recognize the changes if they looked for them. Woods and lakes and farms form a mental picture of a rural alternative, the reassuring sense that one could choose no longer to live in a suburb or city. It is true that the loss of farms means an immediate practical loss of only a few excellent foods. When you lose a dairy farmer, you often lose a maple-syrup producer. Although the rural north country has attracted small producers of berries, apples, lamb, beef, fresh vegetables, poultry, game birds, honey, and cheeses, these recent efforts are few and scattered; most are in fragile economic condition. But as the population grows, surely we will need this northeastern land for farming. Currently, the best valley land is likely to be the first to be developed.

The situation calls to mind the thousands of acres of prime farmland that lie beneath the nation's highways and the industrial and commercial development they eventually attract. In Vermont, anyone can watch the development creep up Interstate 91 from the Massachusetts border year by year. Dennis Kauppila passed on to me the theory that no place within a four-hour radius of a major city is safe from the pressures of second-home building, and he added that former small cities are quickly becoming major. A glance at the map offers no comfort at all.

Certainly, the same changes are occurring in other parts of North America and in Europe, where there is the same influx of second-home buyers and the same erosion of what is best and most distinctive about a place. But how much more compelling when one lives in the midst of the changes.

Farms make rural areas rural. "Rural," reaching back to the pre-Latin roots—the very word means room, space. Farms define agricultural states and counties; they give many of us a large part of the pleasure we get from being in the country. They divide country from city. Having realized that farms were in a more precarious state than I knew, I began to ask myself questions. Are people really living on $11,000 a year? Why do they continue to farm?

I spoke about farm income to farming friends nearby and was invited to talk over drinks the next evening. George Kempton is one of our town's three selectmen. He doesn't come from a farming family, but he attended a small prep school that was on a farm near where he lived in the southern part of the state; as part of the curriculum, the students ran the farm. Later, he worked for sixteen years as a hired man before he had a farm of his own. When I think of him, I remember hearing about the horses the Kemptons had that were never properly "broke" and that they used to ride bareback, sometimes at a gallop. George likes excitement. He farms 400 acres and milks 130 cows, five or six times as many as most farmers milked a generation ago. One married son, Matt, farms with his father and shares in whatever profits are generated by the business. Normally, life doesn't allow for cocktails at an hour when milking should be done, but Matt had taken charge of the farm for a couple of days to give his father time off to hunt. I asked George about those statistics for income. "The numbers sound pretty good." He explained that some farmers are heavily in debt and vulnerable to the first piece of ill luck, while others do all right. "There's an amazing spread. We make a good living farming."

I pressed my question again. People really live on $11,000 a year? "How people can live on that is an interesting thing." The low cash income doesn't include items subsidized by the farm: a portion of electric and telephone bills, wood for heat from the farm woodlot, meat raised and eaten on the farm, milk. "It's always been difficult. I don't think you farm for the money. That's the main thing. You like the life." Despite my demurral, George showed me his farm books for the last three years. I will only say that, although this particular farm appears to thrive, a good living in Vermont isn't anywhere close to a good living in the city.

Of course, as some people point out, cash income doesn't include the value of capital improvements, such as newly acquired land or new buildings and equipment, nor does it include the constantly inflating value of northeastern real estate. But the only way of realizing that income is to sell out, and dare you suggest to certain people that the value of real estate should be considered as income, you may get an angry response. Selling out to developers means the end of farming. How can you call something farm income that puts an end to farming? Once the land is developed, it is destroyed for any future agriculture.

Paul and Kristine Stecker live only a couple of miles from me. They are, respectively, twenty-six and twenty-three. Paul has been working on farms since he was eleven, but the two of them have had their own farm for only a year and a half. Their start-up capital was two cows. Like other farmers, they work fifteen or sixteen hours a day. They're in the barn at three-thirty in the morning to start the first milking and they're in bed at seven at night. While they milked their jersey herd one afternoon, Paul explained that paying off the first five-year note is hardest; after that you qualify for a mortgage at a lower rate. So a young couple just starting out *can* succeed at dairy farming in the northeast? Paul answers, "So far. . . . I don't know." Kristine has been mostly quiet but she says, "By the skin of your teeth." Is the average jersey farmer making $11,568? Paul thinks that "sounds about right." A year ago you heard it couldn't get any worse, but it did. The price of milk went up, but the price of grain went *way* up. Is anybody doing well? "If you're staying in, you're doing well." The Steckers plan to specialize in show cattle and in breeding to supplement the income from milk. Anyway, Paul says, the reason they farm is "the way of life," acknowledging that the phrase is a cliché. "When you have a good day, you have a really good day. Every time I've seen a calf born it's a thrill. In January there's the smell of summer trapped in the hay. . . . There's the good feeling you get in a blizzard when the cows are warm in the barn." And the results of your work—say, mowing a field—are tangible: "You can look back and see what you've done."

I met Norman Gilman at a small slaughterhouse in the nearby town of St. Johnsbury. Norman farms and works part-time at butchering, depending on the season. He lives in the plain brick house where he was born fifty years ago. His graying red hair is thinning and his face is well-wrinkled from the sun. His smile is warm. As far as he knows, none of his forebears did anything but farm, and "That's all I ever done," except for a little butchering. He doesn't wish he had done anything different. He milks about sixty cows ("just kinda keep it agoin' "), with the help of his oldest son, whose main income results from working for the railroad ("He don't really like to do it"). Before too long, the son will have put in ten years with the railroad, so he'll qualify for some retirement benefits and be able to afford to quit. Then he'll farm full-time.

To Norman Gilman, it is important that the family farm continue for its own sake. When I talked to him some months ago, he left me with the impression he wasn't making any money at all. Recently, I spoke to him about farming, and we were both enjoying the conversation so much that I couldn't work it around to ask exactly how difficult the situation was. He did mention that "if you figured out all your time, you don't make much money." Without the rhythm of his speech, his words don't look like much on paper. He farms because: "I like to do it. I like milking cows. I like getting out in the field."

Ironically, almost from the moment of first settlement, decline has been the theme of hill-country agriculture. The moments of general success have been few, though some people have always managed to farm and prosper. In the years before and after 1800, when the wall of the Appalachians held a flourishing population back from the West, many settlers pushed northward. They cleared the northern New England forests, oblivious to erosion or soil improvement; merely to have cleared the land and broken it to the plow increased its value so much that the farmer who cleared the land would sell it to the next comer and start over on a new piece of wilderness. The farms were self-sufficient: a cow, pigs, hay, grain, chickens, a few vegetables, and a horse or ox for work and transportation. When the opportunity arose, many of the most ambitious farmers migrated west; others escaped to city factories looking for a better life. Meanwhile, farms were becoming less self-sufficient, sending beef, dairy products, grain, and wool to market, and buying their goods from city suppliers.

The common specialty, when there was one, was sheep. The high point of sheep raising was reached around 1840, when in

Vermont there were more than a million and a half. The primary product was wool, not meat (for which many farmers felt a distaste). Many upland pastures were cleared. Sheep sometimes displaced humans when neighboring farms were bought up for pasture. Roughly 75 percent of the land was cleared, a proportion since reversed. In a brief moment of naïveté it was believed that the West wasn't suited to sheep; they could only be raised in the cold hills of the East. But New England quickly found it difficult to compete both with the West and, as the protective tariff was gradually lowered, with Australia. By 1850, the number of sheep in Vermont was reduced to half a million.

The Civil War revived the sheep industry, but after the war the price of wool collapsed. And of the soldiers from Maine, New Hampshire, and Vermont who fought in the war, fewer than half came back to live in their home states. Together with western competition, a final reduction of the wool tariff in the 1880s pushed the remaining farmers toward dairy farming; railroads now carried the dairy products to cities. And each farmer began to work a smaller amount of land more intensively. The new horse-drawn machinery couldn't manage steep rough fields, and old high pastures and small stony fields returned to woods. Lesser specialties were found in apples, potatoes, and poultry. Still, farms continued to be abandoned.

In the town where I live, the cow population reached its peak in 1930. A favorable innovation that followed was the tractor. Generally, farmers in northern Vermont switched to tractors in the forties, some as late as the fifties. Most couldn't afford to keep their horses after that unless they worked them in the woods. Animals had to earn their keep.

The late husband of my next-door neighbor was one of the last in town to switch; he bought his first tractor in 1950. Did the tractor make a difference? Earlene Moore answers slowly and with a smile, "Oh, yeah." A tractor required a whole new set of equipment. Hay was baled for the first time. Francis Moore kept his horses for another fifteen years for gathering sap in the maple orchard, which the tractor couldn't manage. He continued to farm until he was seventy-five, for the pleasure of it; he only stopped when he was weakened by an operation, and even then he kept on for a year after Earlene urged him to quit. "He didn't want to stop. He didn't want to sell his cows." She says softly, pausing between words, "He just—liked—cows. He liked the animals. I never saw him strike an animal." She continues, "Farming was never easy. Francis made every acre count. He was a good farmer."

The history books record some hard economic facts, but no one I know remembers the past ruefully. Looking back, the old people recall a time that was happy. (And today they are happy, generous, and kind, though at first they may show a Yankee reserve.) I remember once meeting an older farmer called Junior Brown, who had a local reputation for his skill at slaughtering pigs. One spring afternoon he stopped as he was passing a house that I was building, an activity he tacitly disapproved. As we talked he grew impassioned about the way the country-side used to look in June: well-tended fields, though more of them, with roadsides neatly mowed by scythes. "Everything was green." He stressed and drew out each word as if somehow, could he make the image strong enough in my mind, the past might return.

The interstate highways took away much of the separateness of this place. Today, from the center of the Northeast Kingdom, it is about five and a half hours to New York, three and a half to Boston, two and a half to Montreal. Some Quebecers vacation here. But the entire southern half of Vermont is too close to New York and Boston to escape the disfiguring effects of year-round tourism. Northwestern Vermont has been transformed by the booming economy and rapid development around the city of Burlington on Lake Champlain. The change echoes many miles inland. Elsewhere, development surrounds individual ski areas and the small metropolises of Montpelier (smallest state capital) and Barre (where the old granite quarries are still active). Gradually, the core of the old-style Vermont has been reduced to a portion of the Northeast Kingdom plus a few unregenerate pockets of rusticity elsewhere that are too flat to afford views or that up to now have escaped notice.

Last year, at the end of October, about three weeks after the leaves had fallen, I spent a day driving north along the Connecticut River to look again at those places in the Northeast Kingdom that I knew remained more or less unchanged. Caledonia, Orleans, and Essex counties make a jagged shape, narrow at the bottom and swelling toward the Canadian border. I live in the southern part of this area, about fifty miles from Canada in a straight line. I had hardly left home when I was surprised and disheartened to discover half a dozen new second homes overlooking the Connecticut River, larger than most of the new year-round homes that the rest of us inhabit. These houses had an air of comfort and affluence, even stylishness. Fortunately, I saw nothing else as monied during the rest of the day. Gilman was an antidote, a small mill town, rare in this country. No bad smell from the paper mill, but not a pretty town. Heading north out of town I saw no farms. As if to underline my mood, the day was overcast. And my notes from the trip are appropriately laconic.

I passed a long covered bridge to New Hampshire, two spans. The river was full, slow, and beautiful near the town of Lunenburg, flat fields in both states. On the Vermont side a big dairy farm surrounded a brick Federal-period house. A little farther on was the Country Kettle Restaurant at lunchtime, with many cars parked and three tractor-trailers. I followed the small state highway north with the river. There were both cultivated and abandoned fields. Some farm buildings were put to their intended use; most were used for another purpose, empty, or fallen down. There were more woods than anything else and no traffic. Later, I saw a dozen trucks, including two shiny long-distance milk trucks, but for much of the trip there were no cars on the road.

In Guildhall, the Essex County seat, was the courthouse and a village green lined with clapboarded houses and an old building marked "The Guild Hall." A turn-of-the-century library seemed slightly grand and out of place. Near the virtually nonexistent town of Maidstone, a dead moose lay in the back of a pickup truck in a driveway. Five or six children and teenagers stood around the moose, the children petting the enormous head. It's illegal to shoot this animal in Vermont, and New Hampshire's

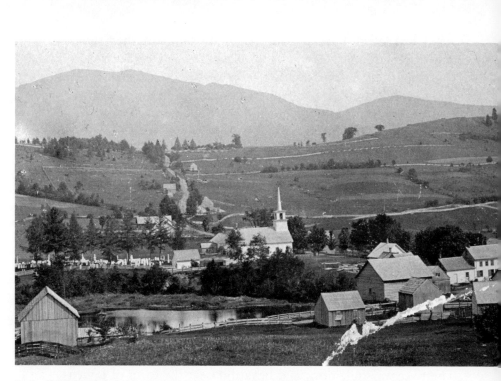

Burke Hollow, Caledonia County, Vermont, before 1896. Photo courtesy of
Mrs. Kenneth Ball.

first season in many years had closed. In Essex County, plenty of
game is shot out of season; quite possibly it was a game
warden's truck.

More miles northward and the valley opened out. Cows were
grazing and the oxbows of the river cut an aimless path through
the fields. The horizontal lines of the level scene recalled a
romantic nineteenth-century painting of an English landscape.
The obvious modern intrusions were the white plastic used to
wrap huge round hay bales that lined the edge of some fields
and the same plastic elsewhere in eight- or ten-foot-wide tubes,
several hundred feet long and filled with silage. The next stretch
of highway had been unpaved the last time I drove it. Here and
there were old and new houses, old and new trailers, a few old
houses that looked abandoned but weren't, the occasional litter

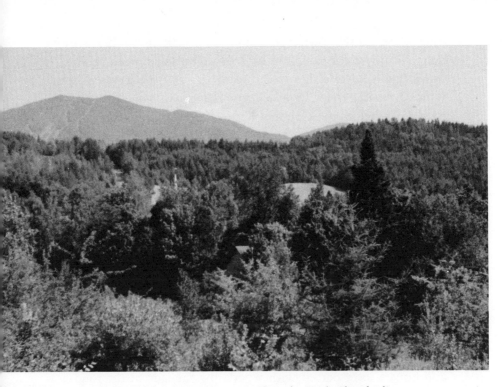

Burke Hollow, Caledonia County, Vermont, 1989. Photo by Keith Chamberlin.

of junked vehicles and farm machinery. Up ahead a dump truck turned onto the highway, ignoring the stop sign.

After a long distance of woods the road looked down on another wide section of valley, more lovely than before: grass still green and marked into flat irregular fields by hedgerows; cows here and there; oxbows of the river again marking a crazy border between the two states; tall New Hampshire mountains behind. Farther on, I passed an old white building the size of a garage, the Brunswick Town House. No village to be seen. The town of Bloomfield did exist, without charm. Columbia Bridge was a covered bridge shorter than the earlier one. A tiny old schoolhouse with shuttered windows: "Town Hall, Leamington, Vt., Chartered 1762." Again, no village.

The land flattened out toward Canada, and there was little of interest before the town of Canaan. South of town a big working dairy farm was for sale, and beyond that a farm recently shut down had a for-sale sign nailed to the barn. A field was planted with Christmas trees. Finally, I saw the first automobiles on the road since before the Country Kettle Restaurant. Canaan proper was fair-sized, with some houses decorated in a Quebec style, more flamboyant than the usual Yankee one. But in late October the land was stark. I turned west and passed through a dozen miles of little more than short fir trees and a pond or two with cottages, before there was open land again, encompassing the town of Norton. There were going farms here, an island of agriculture, but again many fields were abandoned and growing up. Some farms were for sale, including one of the most prosperous-looking. Leaving Norton I had to drive southwest because there is no road along the border. No human habitation, nothing but firs for another dozen miles. Then, I turned onto the first road to the northwest and left Essex County.

The town of Morgan was again hilly and hospitable, farms and houses interspersed with woods. By the side of the road a spring poured out from behind granite blocks. An old Vermont couple had stopped to drink; the man filled two red cups while his wife waited in the car. When I reached the town of Derby, I left the old-style country. There was new commercial development along the highway, the first change I'd seen that looked as if it were fueled by outside stimulus rather than being the modest growth inherent in the local economy. I crossed the edge of the larger town of Newport—more new commercial development. Then I drove onto the interstate and headed home, south through the heart of Orleans County, where there were many views from higher elevations. The rounded hilltops were often still farmed. The highest point on the interstate is 1,856 feet, the divide between the Connecticut and St. Lawrence river valleys. No farms near there nowadays.

There is or was a faint undercurrent of violence in the Northeast Kingdom, left over from the old way of life—hardly threatening, but present. There was never any particular belief that the law was wiser than you were. (Going back fifty years, it was commonly held that the only proper business of government was tending to roads and schools.) I knew a man who, years ago, used to hunt deer jointly with his neighbors; no matter who shot the animal, each hunter in his turn took a deer home to feed his family. They didn't care about hunting seasons. This man sold his farm to a developer in 1971; he left one field half plowed.

Fifteen years ago, there were still old men who never drove faster than twenty or twenty-five miles an hour (their sense of speed conditioned by a horse) and who would nearly always stop for a hitchhiker, probably because people just used to help each other. I've heard people in other parts of the state complain that no one there ever waves anymore. But a friend from Manhattan who comes to visit me here says it makes him uneasy when people automatically make eye contact or when I wave to strangers.

Until recently, the low cost of land and houses helped to compensate for low wages, but now out-of-state incomes are competing with local incomes for real estate. When I first built a house up here, there were no building permits required and no zoning. Now there are too many people, and we no longer put our trust in the benevolence of the free market.

Like other faraway places, the Northeast Kingdom has always seemed to be a refuge. What you did was your business; a measure of independence was the norm. Until recently, people didn't necessarily "work *out*," meaning work off the farm or for someone else. The countryside didn't empty in the morning when people left to work in the larger towns. You expected to see people moving about all day long. But increasingly, rural areas are mainly residential areas, though there are farmers, loggers, perhaps a sawmill or a business repairing small engines, the occasional interloping artist or writer. In the small villages there is usually a store or garage, a library or town clerk's office to provide a semblance of former commercial life. (After all, commerce, not sociability, was the reason the cluster of village houses came into being.)

What does it mean when truly rural places cease to exist near us? Perhaps for many city people, the existence of farms and wilderness was never important to an understanding of the world. But to others it gives a sense of one's proportion in nature, a sense that the built world isn't as all-important as it sometimes appears. To them, nature is a necessary constant. An agricultural countryside also gives an appreciation of where our food comes from (and suggests, I think, how good it can be). After a season in the city the countryside is invigorating. The wilderness suggests unknown possibilities; or at least the absence of wilderness suggests limits.

Despite my lamentations, I still find this place beautiful and different. These are the qualities that make it vulnerable, the reason why people continue to move here. But for the latest comers, no one may drop by to describe how his mother dried her beans for threshing by draping the plants over small fir trees, cut and trimmed for the purpose — as an old fellow once told me while I worked in my garden. The old cooking around here was at best good, plain, hearty food; but to the extent that distinctive regional food develops from stability and tradition, the opportunity for building and improving on it seems to be lost.

Many unfortunate changes have to be accepted. Since 1940, Vermont has lost over 80 percent of its dairy farms. There are about half as many cows today as there were then, but the average cow produces almost three times as much milk. And the agricultural extension service expects that dairy farmers' efficiency will continue to increase, though the demand for dairy products rises only slowly. Greater productivity will put even more farmers out of business. Between January 1988 and January 1989, Vermont lost 6 percent of its milk producers; overall, New England lost 7 percent.

Yet, there are ways to ease the economic pressure on farmers (accepting that it is highly improbable for the price of milk somehow to leap upward). The greatest problem is the basic cost of acquiring farmland. Almost nowhere in the northeast can a dairy farmer buy land and hope to pay for it by selling agricultural products. The situation is nearly impossible for young farmers with little capital just starting out. One excellent solution is to have government or a private organization buy the rights to develop threatened farmland in order to reduce the price of this land to its agricultural worth—as opposed to its value to a developer. The effect is similar to that of zoning, but without confiscating from the farmer his primary investment, the one he is usually counting on for his retirement. The purchase of development rights is a way to permanently protect important agricultural as well as wild areas. But, of course, this takes money, and it is only beginning to have a major effect.

If someone bought the development rights to two of the dairy farms I mentioned at the outset, it would enable a young couple to buy the farm they're renting (the owner believes it is worth $400,000 to a developer), and it would enable an established farm couple to divide the value of their farm fairly among all their children, since only one of them has joined the father in farming.

Why do people farm? "You can't count your hours, or you sink into a mire of depression," says a woman in my town who retired some years ago from farming. "You have to like farming. You have to like working all the time." Of the couple who bought her farm, she says: "They don't want to do anything else."

Two

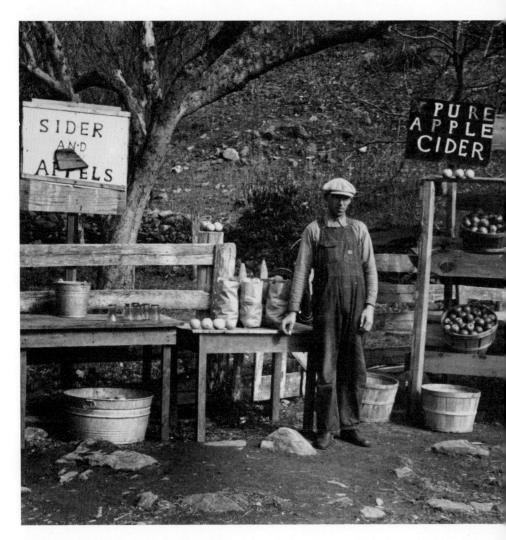

Apple Stand. Photo by Arnold Rothstein.

Paradise Lost: The Decline of the Apple and the American Agrarian Ideal

Anne Mendelson

> The studies of nature have been wisely ordained by Omnip-
> otence as the most pleasing to the mind of man; and it is in
> the unbounded field which natural objects present, that he
> finds that enjoyment which their never-ending novelty is
> peculiarly calculated to impart, and which renders their
> study devoid of that satiety which attaches itself to other
> pursuits. Most wisely has it thus been prescribed, that by an
> occupation of the mind, itself inviting and recreative, we
> should be insensibly led on to a development of the intrica-
> cies of nature, and be thus taught to appreciate the benefi-
> cence of the Creator, by a knowledge of the perfection and
> beauty which mark the labours of his hand.[1]

This exalted tribute sounds for all the world like some minor
Enlightenment philosopher explaining the essential harmony of
religion and natural science. In fact, it is from a manual on successful fruit growing written by a nurseryman in Flushing, New
York, during the administration of Andrew Jackson. It asserts
something that struck chords in many American hearts for

This article is loosely based on an earlier version that formed part of a talk
given by Lee Grimsbo and me to the Culinary Historians of New York in June
1988. I am grateful to Mr. Grimsbo for sharing with me not only important
books but also his wide knowledge of American pomiculture. I have omitted,
with regret, several critical developments in American fruit-growing history.
The most important are the worldwide export trade in American fruit from
about the 1850s into the early twentieth century, the early golden age of
scientific pomology beginning with the establishment of the state agricultural
experiment stations in 1887, and the rise of West Coast fruit farming (with
corresponding loss of eastern production) from about the turn of the century.

several generations: that cultivating an orchard offers intellectual, even spiritual, benefits befitting an enlightened citizenry. True, the writer also noted that the climate and soil of the United States had proved wonderfully suited "to the culture of the various fruits" and that such pursuits "tend greatly to advance the wealth of a community." But what roused him to real eloquence was the delight an orchard yielded to the contemplative mind.

Had William Robert Prince, the author of *The Pomological Manual,* been transported from 1831 to 1914, he would have found the Apple Advertisers of America putting their muscle behind National Apple Day with a campaign including prizes for school essays on apples and free distributions to florists or restaurateurs willing to help plug the product. Getting the public to buy apples, the organization explained in its new publication *The Apple World,* was nothing to be left to chance. "We are finally waking up to the fact that the Apple business is too big, too important, too valuable, to be allowed to drift about on the commercial sea 'the sport and prey of racking whirlwinds.' We must steady its course through selling efficiency made possible by sane and sound publicity methods."[2] The cover depicted a large globelike apple afloat on cosmic clouds, with a map of North America firmly plastered across the center beneath a label reading "The World's Apple Orchard."

In the gap between these two visions of the American orchard lies a story of hope and disillusionment unmentioned in most histories of American agriculture. The twentieth-century end of the story is familiar: a society that wouldn't eat at all if not for steep, risky capital investments on the part of growers continually struggling for a surer hold on markets. But at the other end, close to the birth of the republic, is something we have mostly forgotten: The vast resources of the continent then seemed to promise that ordinary people might not just lead self-sufficient lives on their own land but enjoy a reward that once had been only the pleasure of the rich — an orchard.

Most of us vaguely recall Jefferson's hope to see America a nation of small farmers. It is less widely understood that, even in Jefferson's lifetime, others were refining the plainspun agrarian ideal, to suggest that in a land of equals, the smallest farm should also make room for the finer things of life. Gardens, especially orchards, were longstanding symbols of sheltered leisure and privilege. More recently, they had become the venue for such glamorous attempts to improve on nature as the seventeenth-century tulip mania or the practice of "inoculating" (grafting) fruit trees, deplored in Marvell's poem "The Mower Against Gardens." By the end of the eighteenth century, the luxury of a flower, vegetable, or fruit garden had filtered down more widely to the middle class. So had a conviction that such things, far from being fripperies, were good for the mind and spirit.

We can put together a lively picture of the American orchard idyll and its nineteenth-century fortunes by looking at accounts of orchard fruits—particularly apples—in the wealth of horticultural writing already well established by midcentury. Today we rarely think of classifying fruit and vegetable raising under the rubric of "horticulture" (garden cultivation) as opposed to "agriculture" (field crop raising). But, for some years of our history, the word "horticulture" had a novel sheen, promising an America made happier and more beautiful by the civilizing influence of gardening skill in every rural home.

Nothing seemed to promise more happiness and beauty than the apple. It has always been the American fruit par excellence, partly reflecting an early preference for cider as a beverage. Probably no country on earth offers more extraordinary scope in terms of growing conditions to the genetic possibilities of *Malus pumila,* which throws up a new combination of qualities every time an apple blossom is pollinated. Amelia Simmons's *American Cookery* declared in 1796 that, if every American family had a properly cared-for apple tree, "The net saving would in time extinguish the public debt, and enrich our cookery."[3] This patriotic thought only echoed a widely shared faith in the virtues of fruit raising. Already some of the agricultural societies founded in the eastern states during the eighteenth century were devoting much attention to horticulture; they would soon be supplemented by horticultural and later pomological societies singing the praises of orchards. An early paean from this era was delivered around 1804 by a member of the Kennebec (Maine) Agricultural Society:

> When we consider the various manners in which fruits are beneficial, when we recollect the pleasure they afford to the senses, and the chaste and innocent occupation which they give in their cultivation; when we consider the reputation which they communicate to a country in the eye of strangers, especially as affording a test of its climate and industry; when we remember the importance of improving the beverage which they are intended to supply; when it is calculated under how many solid forms they may be exported (as dried, baked, and preserved, as well as in their natural state;) and lastly, when we reflect upon the utility of giving to our rural labours a thoughtful turn, which is the best substitute we have, after having quitted our primeval state; I say, when we consider these things, it will appear that the subject of fruits, which were the first earthly gift of Providence to man in his more favoured state, may well continue to merit both the publick and individual attention.[4]

James Thacher's 1825 treatise *The American Orchardist,* which approvingly quotes this lofty thought, notes that, "in the whole department of rural economy, there is not a more noble, interesting, and beautiful exhibition, than a fruit orchard, systematically arranged, while clothed with nature's foliage, and decorated with variegated blossoms perfuming the air, or when bending under a load of ripe fruit of many varieties."[5]

One could multiply examples from the early American horticultural literature. Like William Robert Prince, the commentators duly noted the commercial potential of the product. But what is striking today is their moral and aesthetic fervor and the assumption that fruit raising was a pleasure by which any citizen could enrich our common life. That note continued to be sounded as the canals and railroads began opening up more of the continent to cultivation. It was still being sounded late in the nineteenth century. One strain of opinion thought home-scale pomiculture beneficial to the family, viewed by most nineteenth-century writers on domestic affairs as the great moral nurturing ground. In *The American Fruit Culturist* (1849), John Jacob

Thomas declared that the home with an attraction like its own fruit garden had a "salutary bearing" on growing children. John A. Warder's *American Pomology: Apples,* published in 1867, also asserts that a lifetime of happy, improving associations can be stored up through childhood by the delights of the home garden and orchard. Beyond the strengthening of familial ties, Warder thought that planting and taking care of one's own tree was an excellent early lesson in property rights. Fruit stealing was a common symbol of juvenile crime, nineteenth-century style, but this observer saw the cure not in deploring the crime-producing or "sybaritic" effect of "luxuries" like fruit but in letting young children learn about *mine* and *thine* from growing their own. Each would then "appreciate the beauties of the moral code, which he will be all the more likely to respect in every other particular." [6]

An allied claim was that small-scale fruit growing fostered a larger sort of communal unity and stability. The well-known Rochester nurseryman Patrick Barry argued along this line in *The Fruit Garden* (1852). Fruit culture, he announced as a self-evident truth, was an interest linking all classes and occupations from "agriculturist" to "merchant or professional man" and "artizan."

> It is the desire of every man, whatever may be his pursuit or condition in life, whether he live in town or country, to enjoy fine fruits, to provide them for his family, and, if possible, to cultivate the trees in his own garden with his own hands. . . . Fortunately, in the United States, land is so easily obtained as to be within the reach of every industrious man; and the climate and soil being so favorable to the production of fruit, Americans, if they be not already, must become truly "a nation of fruit growers." [7]

Several years before, a farmer named Henry French in Exeter, New Hampshire, had praised the stabilizing effect of apple growing in a letter submitted to the Patent Office for its 1849 agricultural report. (From 1839 until President Lincoln established the Department of Agriculture in 1862, the Patent Office acted as a general clearinghouse of information on all aspects of farming.) French opined:

> An influence is much needed in New England to counterbalance the roving propensity of her people; an influence which is nowhere so surely to be found as in the strengthening of home-ties by the union of labor with the works of nature. He who has planted a tree, will he not desire to eat of the fruit thereof? and he whose father has raised it, will he not feel it to be almost sacrilege to give it into the hands of strangers?
>
> Patriotism has no basis so secure as in the love which man has for his home and the home of his fathers.[8]

The force of this claim cannot be appreciated by casual visitors to a modern orchard. Most apple trees are by nature slow to mature. What Henry French knew as standard apple trees reached spreading heights like twenty or even forty feet and might take from seven to twelve years to start bearing, though they then usually went on for decades. A long-lived, space-hungry orchard like that obviously gave its planters a stake in staying put—something altered in our lifetime not only by urban sprawl but by the practice of grafting virtually all varieties onto dwarfing or semidwarfing rootstocks that reduce the size and life span of the mature tree along with the time it takes to start bearing. (A modern orchard may crop within two or three years.)

If we want an eloquent summary of the inspiration that the nineteenth-century pomologists sought in fruit raising, it is furnished by John Warder in a passage insisting that, for all the importance of agriculture, it is the pursuit of horticulture that "always marks the advancement of a community":

> As our western pioneers progress in their improvements from the primitive log cabins to the more elegant and substantial dwelling houses, we ever find the garden and the orchard, the vine-arbor and the berry-patch taking their place beside the other evidences of progress. These constitute to them the poetry of common life, of the farmer's life.[9]

But the Exeter farmer, noting that New Englanders tended to *leave* New England, had hinted at something already quite unlike the manual writers' picture of the happy home orchard as a bright influence cementing family and community. The fact was that the life regularly painted as American rural destiny had little to do with the actual choices of people living on the land, even in the first heyday of American orchardry. Home orchards indeed there were, for a very long time. One still sees their remnants on old farms in many parts of the Northeast and the Midwest. To travelers, they seemed one of the most characteristic features of the American landscape. Sereno Todd's *The Apple Culturist* (1871) quoted Horace Greeley on the "air of comfort and modest thrift" that such living tokens of refinement gave to a homestead:

> If I were asked to say what single aspect of our economic condition most strikingly and favorably distinguished the people of our Northern States from those of most if not all other countries which I have traversed, I would point at once to the fruit trees which so generally diversify every little as well as larger farm throughout these States, and are quite commonly found even on the petty holdings of the poorer mechanics and workmen in every village, and in the suburbs and outskirts of every city.[10]

These pretty clusters of trees barely hinted at what had happened since the early horticultural cheerleading in the first decades of the century. The fact was that thousands of farmers had been persuaded to invest great amounts of land and money in fruit, especially apples, *as a specialized cash crop*. "The public mind has waked up to the importance of this subject, and in some sections is roused even to a sort of enthusiasm upon it," a Massachusetts contributor to the 1849 Patent Office report sanguinely noted.[11] Three years later, in *The Fruit Garden,* Patrick Barry grandly pooh-poohed those who thought the fruit-growing craze "a sort of speculative mania."[12] Ominous realities were masked by this optimism. The true story of nineteenth-century pomiculture is how the business of producing apples for a market assumed a demanding, risky life of its own even as charming tributes to home orchardry filled the pages of manuals and journals. We see the two unfolding together in the preface of the foremost pomological manual of the century, A. J. Downing's *Fruits and Fruit Trees of America,* first published in 1845 and issued in many revisions until 1896:

> America is a *young orchard,* but when the planting of fruit-trees in one of the newest States numbers nearly a quarter of a million in a single year; when there are more peaches exposed in the markets of New York, annually, than are raised in all France; when American apples, in large quantities, command double prices in European markets; there is little need for entering into any praises of this soil and climate generally, regarding the culture of fruit. In one part or another of the Union every man may, literally, sit under his own vine and fig tree.[13]

The vine-and-fig-tree model was just what the early horticulturists had preached as a fit image of rural America. But it was not consistent with the vision of orchards as gold mines. Downing's claims about European prices for American apples and the New York markets' selling more peaches than the entire output of France, at a time when hopeful investors were putting in a quarter of a million fruit trees in *one* new state alone, suggest a widespread rush to make a buck. It was a dangerous game even then, for circumstances that would be minor disappointments or even blessings to the self-sufficient rural family with a plot of fruit trees were absolute catastrophes to a farmer who had staked all on a large orchard.

One occasion of rude awakening was the seasonal glut of the market, still worse in years of bumper crops. This was, ironically, the consequence of living in a peerless region for raising apples. At the time of the initial fruit-growing boom—the last twenty or thirty years before the Civil War—growers competing with dozens or hundreds of others for city fruit markets could do little to store apples more than a few weeks, except for varieties like Winesap that naturally kept well over the winter. Some of the best dessert apples, articles that commanded glamorous prices in the cities, were fragile and short-lived, not easy to get to market in good condition under the best circumstances. (The Fameuse or Snow apple, thought to be a parent of the McIntosh, was one of these difficult beauties.) Another problem was the biennial tendency of some popular varieties including Baldwin, Roxbury Russet, and Northern Spy, which might bear handsomely one year and hardly at all the next.

Turning large tracts of land in New England, New York, and the upper Midwest into fruit orchards had another effect: It created ideal habitats for insect scourges that had been less devastating in a time of scattered, nonintensive fruit cultivation. These pests now assumed dire economic significance. From the early boom in the 1830s until near the end of the century, orchardists regularly lost whole crops (or large percentages) to insects. The nineteenth-century growth of the city "fancy trade," which paid premium prices but required cosmetically attractive fruit, made even slightly blemished apples less acceptable than they had been before the rise of commercial orchardry. For many years farmers were essentially helpless against insect damage, though they continually wrote to the horticultural journals with tips like the mixture of whale oil soapsuds and tobacco water tried by many against a weevil called the plum curculio, which also relished apples. One reader of A. J. Downing's celebrated magazine *The Horticulturist* reported in 1847 that he had "found that the worm would live after having been immersed in tobacco water so strong as to be as dark as port wine."[14]

The solution to this problem did not appear until the 1880s, when the first effective pesticides applied by spraying were introduced and at once became one of the unavoidable fixed costs of the orchard business. Effective storage was another expensive boon. Neither ice cooling (for which there was fairly good technology from the 1850s and 1860s) nor mechanical refrigeration (well advanced by the last decades of the century) was feasible for most growers to use on their own farms. It was primarily merchants and distributors who would profit from these advances in storage, which incidentally jacked up the cost of getting the fruit from farmer to consumer.

Almost as soon as the big commercial fruit-raising push had reached the northern states, it was obvious that many people had not landed themselves in the vine-and-fig-tree life or in a fountain of riches. From the viewpoint of modern connoisseurs, the scramble for a competitive edge had at least one attractive upshot. This was the great proliferation of apple varieties, something that would not have been possible during the centuries when most apple trees were chance seedlings and only a few hobbyists were interested in "inoculation." (No apple variety can be truly propagated by anything except grafting or budding— "inoculating," as these practices usually were known until the nineteenth century.) A few dozen new American varieties had been propagated, mostly in New York and New England, during the eighteenth century. At least two of these—the Esopus Spitzenburg and the Newtown Pippin—continued to be regarded as the absolute top of the line until well past 1900. But the nineteenth century saw a virtual deluge of new varieties. Suddenly the immense genetic variability of the species was understood as an opportunity for profitable experiment. Already in 1852 Patrick Barry estimated the number of cultivated apple varieties to be at least a thousand, though he chose only 150 for mention in *The Fruit Garden.*

From the 1830s and 1840s on, orchardists developed periodic enthusiasms for some new wonder apple. The Northern Spy and the Jonathan were early sensations that happen to be among the best-flavored apples anywhere on the planet. But good flavor was not the prime consideration of everyone who watched a new seedling for signs of promise and added it to the flood of propagated varieties. Though Barry counted "every [variety] of *real excellence* as an additional blessing to the fruit growers and to society, for which they should be duly grateful,"[15] these blessings were not equally shared among all growers. An apple touted as a miracle in central Connecticut might be mediocre or almost ungrowable in Ohio, Michigan, or western New York. A farmer might find this out after an investment of ten years' time and dozens of acres newly carved from wilderness. Of the literally thousands of varieties grown on some scale during the nineteenth century, only a few dozen proved to have wide commercial potential, and their survival did not necessarily depend on quality. By the end of the Civil War, many growers saw great merit in so-so apples with some particular selling point like size, bright color, smooth skin, inoffensive sweetness, highly reliable cropping, toughness and transportability, or timing to hit the dead spots of the seasonal market.

Some canny observers shortly began to think that the future belonged to a pomiculture based on *fewer* kinds of apples, not more. (It hardly needs saying that they were right. Today most Americans have never seen more than seven or ten varieties of apple, while some like Baldwin and Greening, considered mediocre a century ago, are now head and shoulders above most of what we get.) An orchardist named Seth Fenner, who delivered a paper to an audience of western New York fruit growers in Oswego in 1886, saw quite correctly that the great wealth of apple varieties then being cultivated was a mistaken route to the sacred purpose of making money. "The one great mistake of American orchards," he philosophized, "is the multiplicity of varieties. Multiplicity of varieties work as great damage to orchards as polygamy does to the Mormons, and you want to avoid it. Select a few standard varieties, especially for market."[16] He suggested a list of nine practical choices that entirely omitted the four great glories of New York apple growing—Newtown Pippin, Esopus Spitzenburg, Northern Spy, and Jonathan.

Well into the orchard gold rush, some observers were putting the best face on what had developed into a grinding struggle for many. Allen W. Dodge, the Massachusettsan who had hailed the fruit-growing boom in the 1849 Patent Office report, clearly had heard apprehensive assessments in some quarters. "Suffice it to say, it is no speculative or visionary scheme," he insisted, "but a safe and permanent investment that will yield golden dividends, so long as our soil and seasons shall continue to be as propitious as they have heretofore been." Scorning suggestions by those of "narrow vision" that the market would soon be glutted, he added in a footnote that, anyhow, the prospects of the European market for American fruit were limitless.[17] Patrick Barry's *Fruit Garden* enumerated still more promises of great things to come:

At one time apples were grown chiefly for cider; now they are considered indispensable articles of food. The finer fruits, that were formerly considered as luxuries only for the tables of the wealthy, are beginning to take their place among the ordinary supplies of every man's table; and this taste must grow from year to year, with an increased supply. Those who consume a bushel of fruit this year, will require double or treble that quantity next. The rapid increase of population alone, creates a demand to an extent that few people are aware of. The city of Rochester has added 20,000 to her numbers in ten years. Let such an increase as this in all our cities, towns, and villages be estimated, and see what an aggregate annual amount of new customers it presents.

New markets are continually presenting themselves and demanding large supplies. New and more perfect modes of packing and shipping fruits, and of drying, preserving, and preparing them for various purposes to which they have not hitherto been appropriated, are beginning to enlist attention and inquiry.[18]

Dodge and Barry were right in predicting a vast expansion of markets through new consumption patterns, European exports, experimental technology, and sheer population growth. They were wrong in thinking that gluts could not occur or that an expanded orchard capacity could easily surmount any market vagaries. In some ways the future was bright for American orchardry. It was not bright for the self-sufficient family-scale idyll that continued to be widely depicted as American rural life. The reality of the situation appears much more clearly a dozen-odd years later, in an article on horticulture contributed by an observer named M. L. Dunlop to the transactions of the Illinois State Agricultural Society for 1865–66:

When we take a view of the great variety of agricultural products, we can come to no other conclusion than that it must needs have a division of labor similar to that of the mechanic arts. The farmer may raise grain and cattle and fruits and garden vegetables for market, but when he attempts them all on an even scale, he will make a signal failure. He must choose one of these as the main business, and make the others only secondary, to be pursued as convenient. This is becoming a well settled principle in rural economy, and the true one. We have grain farmers, dairymen, stock-growers, hog-raisers, orchardists, and market-gardeners. . . .

We have reached that point in our progress that the demand for horticultural products is of such a nature that a large part of our rural population and capital can be most profitably employed in it. The demands from our manufacturing cities and marts of commerce must be supplied. But we now have new demands upon us—the railways have opened up to us new markets, and we can send the products of the orchard to the miners of the Rocky Mountains, and the regions of the more inhospitable North.[19]

The change was upon the farmers of the eastern and midwestern fruit-growing regions before anyone had grasped its implication: What had been the pleasurable and spiritually rewarding pursuit of horticulture as a blessing of democracy would have to become just another branch of a very specialized, professionalized, segmented American agricultural economy in which no effort was free of real financial risk. The farmer must decide not what he wanted to grow but what he wanted to sell.

This candid recommendation of specialized fruit farming is a long way from William Robert Prince's praising orchardry as a refreshment for mind and soul. The second great spurt in American pomiculture—ushered in by real scientific advances in pomology around 1890 and lasting until after World War I— would travel even further from the visions of plenty, equality, and enlightenment once conjured up by the thought of raising one's own fruit. Even in the 1860s and 1870s, unhappy accounts of growers' tribulations suggest that what many were really casting about for was the promised cure-all hailed in 1914 by *The Apple World*—advertising, a kind of camshaft linking the crop in the orchards with desired levels of consumption.

Today, tasting the wretched apples from a supermarket or touring an irrigated factory-scale orchard, one can scarcely imagine that people ever attached moral or spiritual value to such things. And in hindsight it is clear that the Eden seen in the American orchard by the horticultural manual writers never really existed. But there is another postscript to the story of fruit growing as part of the early American democratic vision.

In a sense, something that can be called the humanist side of fruit raising never really died out. It was kept alive by some pomologists well into the age of marketing pitches. In 1922 the great horticultural writer Liberty Hyde Bailey commented that a current industry campaign "to lead the people to eat an apple a day" was beside the mark: "To eat an apple a day is a question of affections and emotions." He meant not trivially manipulated preferences but the real inner loyalty to ideals of excellence that distinguished "a good amateur interest in fruits."[20] Seven years before, the same observer had sadly noted what he saw as a true cultural loss:

> It is much to be desired that the fruit-garden shall return to men's minds, with its personal appeal and its collections of many choice varieties, even the names of which are now unknown to the fruit-loving public. . . . The commercial market ideals have come to be controlling, and most fruit-eaters have never eaten a first-class apple or pear or peach, and do not know what such fruits are; and the names of the choice varieties have mostly dropped from the lists of nurserymen. All this is as much to be deplored as a loss of standards of excellence in literature and music, for it is an expression of a lack of resources and a failure of sensitiveness.[21]

Bailey was more right than he could have foreseen about the dismal effect of "commercial market ideals" on the quality of American fruit. But, since he wrote, many thousands of people have done much to justify his regard for "the amateur, who, as the word means, is the lover."[22] For some decades of this century, the fruit-growing tradition found its best American expression in generations of Italian and Middle Eastern immigrants who would no more have been without fruit trees in the smallest yard than without shoes or a roof. And, in the last few decades, another constituency has begun restoring something that belongs to all of us by searching out "heirloom" varieties of apple —

sometimes obscure local specialties—unknown to commercial orchardry for fifty or eighty years. There are enough of these
Quixotes seeking the poetry of common life to be recognized as
a market by some of the largest commercial nurseries. As a
result, the outfits that supply the big growers with the makings
of edible sawdust now also offer home orchardists an increasing
selection of apples fit for William Robert Prince's "occupation of
the mind, in itself inviting and recreative." With no idea on earth
except to enjoy a heritage of excellence first developed on American soil and linked with one of the better American aspirations,
hobbyists are bringing back to life apples like Fameuse, Swaar,
Wagener, Esopus Spitzenburg, Roxbury Russet, and Westfield
Seek-No-Further. There is something in this effort that tran-
scends mere hobby. It keeps alive a loyalty to a younger America
that Professor Bailey understood sixty-seven years ago when he
called the pomological amateur "the embodiment of the best in
the common life, the conservator of aspirations, the fulfillment
of democratic freedom."[23]

Notes

1. William Robert Prince, with William Prince, *The Pomological Manual*
(New York: T. and J. Swords, 1831), p. vii.
2. *The Apple World: The Official Organ of the Apple Advertisers of
America* 1, no. 1 (June 1914), p. 10.
3. Amelia Simmons, *American Cookery* (Hartford, Conn.: Hudson &
Goodwin, 1796), p. 16.
4. Quoted in James Thacher, *The American Orchardist* (Boston: E. Collier,
1825), pp. 14–15.
5. Ibid., p. 11.
6. John A. Warder, *American Pomology: Apples* (New York: Orange Judd,
1867), pp. 14–15.
7. P[atrick] Barry, *The Fruit Garden* (New York: Scribners, 1852), p. iii.
8. Henry F. French, "Cultivation of Apples in the Northern States," in
Report of the Commissioner of Patents for the Year 1849 (Washington, D.C.:
U.S. Patent Office, 1850), pp. 273–76.
9. Warder, *American Pomology*, p. 14.
10. Horace Greeley, quoted in Sereno Todd, *The Apple Culturist* (New York:
Harper & Bros., 1871). pp. 12–13.
11. Allen W. Dodge, "Orchards—Their Condition and Management," in
Report of the Commissioner of Patents for the Year 1849 (Washington, D.C.:
U.S. Patent Office, 1850), p. 276.
12. Barry, *Fruit Garden*, p. iv.
13. A. J. Downing, *The Fruits and Fruit Trees of America* (New York: Wiley

& Putnam, 1845), pp. v–vi.

14. *The Horticulturist and Journal of Rural Art and Rural Taste* 1, no. 9 (March 1847), p. 310.

15. Barry, *Fruit Garden,* p. 278.

16. "Hints to Fruit Growers, Delivered at Oswego Institute, 1886, by Hon. Seth Fenner, of Erie County," in *Transactions of the New York State Agricultural Society* 34 (1883–1886), pp. 200–4.

17. Dodge, "Orchards–Their Condition and Management," pp. 277, 277n.

18. Barry, *Fruit Garden,* p. v.

19. From M. L. Dunlop, "The Status of Horticulture," in *Illinois State Agricultural Society, Transactions, 1865–66,* excerpted in Wayne D. Rasmussen, ed., *Agriculture in the United States: A Documentary History* 2 (New York: Random House, 1975), p. 1053.

20. L. H. Bailey, *The Apple-Tree* (New York: Macmillan, 1922), p. 76.

21. L. H. Bailey, *The Principles of Fruit-Growing, with Applications to Practice* (New York: Macmillan, 1915), p. 35.

22. Bailey, *Apple-Tree,* p. 77.

23. Ibid.

Food, Health, and Native-American Agriculture

Gary Paul Nabhan

"It was this way, long time ago," the old Indian lady—a member of Arizona's Sand Papago tribe that calls itself the O'odham— explained through a distant relative, who was translating: "The People were like a cultivated field producing after its kind, recognizing its kinship; the seeds remain to continue to produce. Today all the bad times have entered the People, and they [the O'odham] no longer recognize their way of life. The People separated from one another and became few in number. Today all the O'odham are vanishing."[1]

Candelaria Orosco sat in a small clapboard house in the depressed mining town of Ajo, Arizona, recalling the native foods that she had hunted, gathered, and farmed before the turn of the century. Her leg hurt her, for the sores on it were taking a long time to heal. Today this is a common affliction of her people, the O'odham, who now suffer from the highest incidence of diabetes of any ethnic population in the world.[2] Orosco was trying hard to describe the life of her kin, the Sand Papagos, as they had lived prior to such afflictions, when they had obtained their living from what outsiders consistently regard as a "hopeless desert." Around the time of Orosco's birth, a U.S. Indian agent had visited the O'odham and described their habitat in this way: "Place the same number of whites on a barren, sandy desert such as they live on, and tell them to subsist there; the probability is that in two years they would become extinct."[3]

Yet, when I spoke to Orosco, she invoked a litany of plant and animal names in her native language; these names refer to herbs and seeds and roots, birds and reptiles and mammals that once formed the bulk of her diet. Even when English rather than O'odham words are used for these nutritional resources, the names of the native food that once filled her larder still have an exotic ring to them. For meat, her family ate desert tortoises, pack rats, bighorn sheep, tomato hornworm larvae, desert cottontails, pronghorn antelope, Gambel's quail, mule deer, white-wing doves, Gila River fish, black-tailed jackrabbits, and occasional stray livestock. Although the unpredictability of desert rains kept her people from harvesting crops on a regular basis at too many places, they did successfully cultivate white tepary beans, Old Lady's Knees muskmelons, green-striped cushaw squash, sixty-day-flour corn, Spanish watermelons, white Sonora wheat, and Papago peas. Perhaps the variety of wild plant foods gathered by her family is more bewildering: broomrape stalks, screwbean mesquite pods, plantain seed, tansy mustard, amaranth, cholla cactus buds, honey mesquite, povertyweed, wolfberries, hog potato, lamb's-quarters, prickly pears, ironwood seed, wild chilies, chia, organ-pipe, senita, and sandfood.[4] When Orosco mentioned the latter plant—an underground parasite that attaches to the roots of wind-beaten shrubs on otherwise barren dunes—my facial expression must have given me away.

"What's that?" she asked in O'odham.

I stammered, "Sandfood . . . did you mean that the old people knew how to find it, and they once told you how it tasted?" Few people alive today have ever seen this sandfood, let alone tasted it, for it is now endangered by habitat destruction.

"I said that *I* ate it. I wouldn't have told you that it had a good sweet taste if I hadn't eaten it myself. How could I explain to you what other people thought it tasted like or how to harvest it? Because it doesn't stick up above the ground like other plants, I had to learn to see where the little dried-up ones from the year before broke the surface. That's where I would dig."

As she described how to steam succulent plants in earthen pits, boil down cactus fruit into jam or syrup, roast meat over an open fire, and parch wild legume seeds to keep them for later use, Orosco spoke matter-of-factly of the work involved in desert subsistence. There were no smackings of romanticism about the halcyon days of her youth; nonetheless, it was clear that she felt some foods of value had been lost. Her concerns about the loss of gathering and farming traditions are much the same as those voiced by her fellow tribesman, the late Miguel Velasco, in an interview with Fillman Bell in 1979:

> We are from the sand, and known as Sand Indians, to find our way of life on the sand of the earth. That is why we go all over to seek our food to live as well. We cover a large portion of land in different harvest seasons to gather our food to store in time of winter season. Long time ago, this was our way of life. We did not buy food. We worked hard to gather foods. We never knew what coffee was until the White People came. We drank the desert fruit juices in harvest time. The desert food is meant for the Indians to eat. The reason so many Indians die young is because they don't eat their desert food. . . . They will not know how to survive if Anglos stopped selling their food. The old Indians lived well with their old way of life.[5]

Nonetheless, oral accounts such as these are often simply dismissed as "nostalgia for the old ways," even by eminent ethnobotanists such as Peter Raven, who used this phrase to introduce a critique of my recent book on Native American agricultural change, *Enduring Seeds*.[6] If we use a simple dictionary definition of "nostalgia"—a longing for experiences, things, or acquaintances belonging to the past—we may or may not include under its rubric some of the statements made by Indian elders. Consider, for instance, this commentary by Chona, recorded by Ruth Underhill in *Autobiography of a Papago Woman* during the early thirties:

> We always kept gruel in our house. It was in a big clay pot that my mother had made. She ground up seeds into flour. Not wheat flour—we had no wheat. But all the wild seeds, the good pigweed and the wild grasses. . . . Oh, how good that gruel was! I have never tasted anything like it. Wheat flour makes me sick. I think it has no strength. But when I am weak, when I am tired, my grandchildren make me a gruel out of the wild seeds. That is *food*.[7]

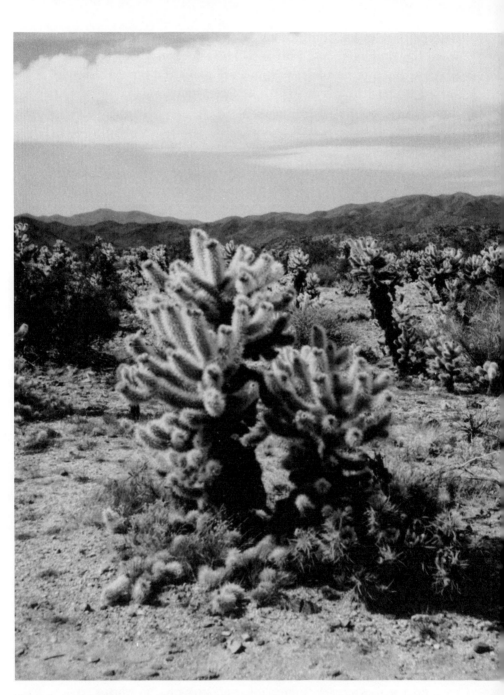

Photo by Will Murphy.

Chona was clearly referring to foodstuffs that had formed a greater proportion of her dietary intake in the past than they did at the time she spoke with Underhill. And yet these foods were not exclusively relegated to the past, because they retained their functional value when she was sick, providing her with nourishment that mainstream American foods could not. Moreover, in Chona's mind, the native desert seeds had remained as the quintessential foods, embodying her cultural definition of what food *should be*. Because she did not consider the value of her people's traditional diet to be obsolete, Chona's respect for that diet should not be relegated to the shelf of antiquarian trivia.

This point was again brought home to me by Candelaria Orosco. After we spent several hours looking at pressed herbs, museum collections of seeds, and historic photos of plants that I had presumed to be formerly part of her culture's daily subsistence, she brought out several of her own collections. She rolled out from under her bed two green-striped cushaw squashes that she had grown in her postage-stamp-sized garden. Then she reached under her stove and showed me caches of cholla cactus buds and some wild seeds she had gathered. These foodstuffs were not simply for "old times' sake"; they had been the fruits of her efforts toward self-reliance for more than ninety years.

Pessimists or self-described "realists" might still dismiss the relict consumption of native foods by Chona or Candelaria Orosco as nostalgic and trivial. Because these plants and animals now make up such a small portion of the diet of contemporary Indians, they are said to play no significant functional role in their nutrition or their culture. If a Navajo eats more Kentucky Fried Chicken than he does the mutton of Navajo-Churro sheep, is it not true that, ecologically and nutritionally speaking, he is more like an urban Kentuckian than he is like his Dine ancestors?

The answer may be a qualified yes. I interpret many of the O'odham elders' statements as warnings to their descendants that they are indeed abandoning what it means to be culturally and ecologically O'odham. This concern is explicit in the following quote from the late great O'odham orator Venito García:

The way life is today, what will happen if the Anglos discontinued their money system? What will happen to our children? They will not want to eat the mountain turtle, because they have never eaten any. Maybe they will eat it if they get hungry enough. I think of all the desert plants we used to eat, the desert spinach we cooked with chile. . . . If we continue to practice eating our survival food, we may save our money we do receive sometimes. . . . The Chinese, they still practice their old eating habits. They save all their money. The Anglos don't like this. They [the Chinese] like to eat their ant eggs [rice]. They even use their long sticks to eat with, picking the ant eggs up with their long sticks and pinning it to their mouths. This is their way of life.[8]

The argument stated so clearly by García is that other cultures have persisted with culinary traditions in a way that is not dismissed as nostalgic conservatism. To be Chinese is to be one who eats rice with chopsticks, according to García's view as an outsider; likewise, an outsider should be able to recognize the desert-dwelling O'odham by their consumption of cactus, amaranth greens, or mesquite. Although such dietary definitions are too restrictive for anthropologists to take seriously, traditional peoples often revealingly use culinary customs as primary indicators of a particular culture.

A further connection is made by O'odham elders in relation to their culinary traditions, and that is their linkage with health and survival. The elders not only recall "survival foods" used during times of drought and political disruption, but they also remember the curative quality of the native foods that were a customary component of their diets. These presumed curative qualities are now being scientifically investigated, for, in a very real sense, native foods may indeed be the best medicine available to the O'odham. The O'odham metabolism evolved under the influence of native desert plant foods with peculiar characteristics that formerly protected the people from certain afflictions now common among them.

Through the thirties, native desert foods contributed a significant portion of Pima and Papago diets; mesquite, chia, tepary beans, cacti, and cucurbits were eaten as commonly as foods introduced by Europeans. At that time, the O'odham were generally regarded as lean, modest people who worked hard at obtaining a subsistence from one of the most unpredictable but biologically diverse deserts in the world. Then government work projects and World War II came along and, rather than tilling their own floodwater fields and small irrigated patches, the O'odham became cheap labor for extensive irrigated cotton farms in Anglo communities near their reservations. Others went off to the war and became accustomed to a cash economy and canned food.

When these people returned to their villages in the late forties, their fields were overgrown or eroded owing to lack of constant care, and off-reservation opportunities were still calling. Government advisers termed their ancient farming strategies risky and unproductive and offered no assistance in renovating the fields that for centuries had remained fertile under periodic cultivation.[9] Instead, the tribal governments were encouraged either to develop their own large farms using the corporate model or to lease tribal lands to non-Indian farmers to do the same. Less than a tenth of the traditional farms of the O'odham survived these economic and social pressures. As the fifties came and went, subsistence farming ceased to be a way of life, while hunting and gathering remained activities for only a small percentage of the indigenes.

Before the war, diabetes had been no more common among the O'odham than it was among the population of the United States as a whole. And yet, twenty-five years later, the O'odham had a prevalence of diabetes fifteen times that of the typical American community. The average young O'odham man in the early 1970s weighed ten pounds more than his 1940s counterpart and was considered overweight verging on obesity. Since obesity is correlated with susceptibility to diabetes, pathologists at first concluded that the "escape" of the O'odham from their primitive, feast-or-famine cycle of subsistence had made calories more regularly available year-round; hence, they had gained weight and diabetes had set in.

The only flaw in this theory was that the modern wage-earning O'odham individual was not necessarily consuming any more calories than his or her traditional O'odham counterpart or, for that matter, than the average Arizona Anglo. The difference, I believe, was not in the number of calories consumed but in the kinds of cultivated and wild plants with which the O'odham had coevolved.

Recently, I sent a number of desert foods traditionally pre- pared by the O'odham to a team of Australian nutritionists, who analyzed the foods for any effects they might have on blood- sugar levels following meals.[10] High blood-sugar levels are of concern because they stress the pancreas. If stressed repeatedly, the pancreas essentially becomes poisoned. Insulin metabolism becomes permanently damaged, and the dangerous syndrome known as diabetes develops. Yet, when a person is fed acorns, mesquite pods, and tepary or lima beans, the special dietary fiber in these foods reduces blood-sugar levels or at least prolongs the period over which sugar is absorbed into the blood. In short, these native foods may protect Indian diabetics from suffering high blood-sugar levels following a meal. Mes- quite pods and acorns are among the 10 percent most effective foods ever analyzed for their effects in controlling blood-sugar rises after a meal.[11]

Other recent studies suggest that many desert foods contain mucilaginous polysaccharide gums that are viscous enough to slow the digestion and absorption of sugary foods. These mucilages have probably evolved in many desert plants to slow water loss from the seeds, seedlings, and succulent tissues of mature plants. The O'odham metabolism may, in turn, have adapted to their qualities after centuries of dependence on them. Prickly pear fruit and pads, cholla cactus buds, plantain seeds, chia seeds, mesquite pods, and tansy mustard seeds contain such gums. All were former seasonal staples of the O'odham; all are nearly absent from their diet today. Australian nutritionist Jennie Brand hypothesizes that these foods served to protect indigenous people from the diabetic syndrome to which they were geneti- cally susceptible.[12]

For those on a traditional diet, diabetes was not likely to be expressed. But diabetes-prone Indians on a fast-food diet of fried potatoes, soft drinks or beer, sweets, and corn chips find their insulin metabolism going haywire. At the Phoenix Indian Hospital, Boyd Swinburn has recently compared the responses of twenty-two patients who changed from a reconstructed, traditional O'odham diet to a fast-food diet consisting of virtually the same number of calories. When they switched to what we nicknamed the "Circle-K diet," their insulin sensitivity to glucose worsened, as did their glucose tolerance. As Swinburn concluded, "The influence of westernization on the prevalence of type 2 diabetes may in part be due to changes in diet composition."[13] For the O'odham and other recently westernized indigenous peoples, a return to a diet similar to their traditional one is no nostalgic notion; it may, in fact, be a nutritional and survival imperative.

In desert villages where native food plants were formerly sown and gathered, the majority of the residents are now classified as unemployed or underemployed. Because their income levels are so low, they are eligible for government surplus commodity foods, nearly all of which have been shown to be nutritionally inferior to their native counterparts.[14] At the same time, the hyperabundance of these federally donated foodstuffs serves as a disincentive for local food production. As one O'odham woman lamented, "Why grow our different kinds of beans when someone delivers big bags of pinto beans to our house every month?" The demise of local farming and gathering, indulgence in a welfare economy, and a worsening of health and self-esteem are linked. This syndrome is not restricted to the O'odham; because of its high Mexican and Indian population, Arizona will by the year 2000 spend $2 billion annually on medical care for its quarter of a million diabetics.[15]

Is it not ironic that, at the same time, more than a quarter-million agricultural acres in Arizona have been abandoned owing to excessive irrigation costs of producing water-consumptive, conventional crops? Native crops, some of which require a third to a fifth as much water as conventional crops to obtain the same economic yield, were not until recently even considered a feasible option.[16] The predominantly Anglo society to which the food industry caters is simply not accustomed to the tastes, textures, and preparation techniques associated with these pre-Columbian foods.

I am reminded of the words of ethnobotanist Melvin Gilmore, who began his work among Indian farmers and gatherers seventy years ago, before the tide of diabetes and agricultural desolation had swamped them:

> We shall make the best and most economical use of our land when our population shall become adjusted in habit to the natural conditions. The country cannot be wholly made over and adjusted to a people of foreign habits and tastes. There are large tracts of land in America whose bounty is wasted because the plants that can be grown on them are not acceptable to our people. This is not because the plants are not useful and desirable but because their value qualities are not known. . . . The adjustment of American consumption to American conditions of production will bring about greater improvement in conditions of life than any other material agency.[17]

If such a call for the return of the native seems to be an affliction of those of us preoccupied with the obscure scholarly pursuit of ethnobotany, perhaps it is pertinent to hear the same call echoed a few years ago by one of America's finest immigrant food writers, Angelo Pellegrini:

> Since Walt Whitman sounded his barbaric yawp over the rooftops of the world, the American landscape has undergone considerable change. The pastoral plains have been impoverished; many of the forests have been denuded; much of the subterranean treasure has been wastefully extracted. The builders of the nation, bold and reckless and impatient, have indeed used the body of America irreverently. . . . And yet, in an exhausted world, America remains a land of plenty. It is no exaggeration to say that its agricultural possibilities are relatively unlimited. . . . An immediate and urgent problem for the American of today is how to use them toward humane living.[18]

As I have written elsewhere, "We will have missed the point if we only select one of these profitable natives, create new hybrids with it, and grow them as monocultures just like any conventional cash crop. The Native American agricultural legacy is more than a few hardy, tasty cultigens waiting to be 'cleaned up' genetically for consumers, and then commercialized as novelty foods. Our goal must be something beyond blue corn chips, tepary bean party dips, amaranth candy, sunflower seed snacks, and ornamental chiles. These nutritious crops deserve to be revived as mainstays of human diets, and not treated as passing curiosities. These cultivated foods are rich in taste and nutrition, yes, but they are also well adapted to the peculiarities of our land."[19]

And the peculiarities of the Native American metabolism may be well adapted to these plant foods. Would it not be less costly to subsidize the revival of native food production and consumption among the O'odham and other diabetes-prone Indians than to assume that an annual $2 billion for health care is an inescapable conclusion? Would it not be better to market native foods grown and gathered by native peoples than to appropriate from them the cream of the crop, only to patent, trademark, privatize, and price them out of the reach of most native peoples? This dilemma has already arisen with wild rice and blue corn: Market prices for elite consumers have driven these native foods beyond a price thought reasonable by many Indian consumers.

And yet certain natives have responded by forming collectives to ensure that some portion of the supplies of these native foods does reach their own people. The Navajo Family Farm project in Leupp, Arizona, and the Ikwe Marketing Collective in White Earth, Minnesota, are but two examples of Native Americans funneling a greater abundance of traditional grains back into their own communities.[20]

Not all the seeds that formerly nourished Native Americans have vanished. Some may have fallen dormant from infrequent usage, but that does not mean that their production cannot be revived. And revival itself is not necessarily a nostalgic cop-out, a retreat from the supposed inexorable trend of dominant societies to make every place, every people, and every meal like all the others. The diminishment of diversity—cultural, culinary, or other—is not inexorable. Ultimately, such diversity may be the soundest means our species has to survive.

Notes

1. Candelaria Orosco interview in Fillman Bell, Keith Anderson, and Yvonne G. Stewart, *The Quitobaquito Cemetery and Its History* (Tucson: Western Archaeological Center, National Park Service, 1980), p. 50.

2. W. C. Knowler, P. H. Bennett, R. F. Hamman, and M. Miller, "Diabetes Incidence and Prevalence in Pima Indians: A 19-fold Greater Incidence than in Rochester, Minnesota," *American Journal of Epidemiology* 108 (1978), p. 497.

3. E. A. Howard, an 1887 Indian agent at the Pima Agency, quoted in G. P. Nabhan, "Papago Indian Desert Agriculture and Water Control in the Sonoran Desert, 1697–1934," *Applied Geography* 6 (1986), pp. 43–59.

4. Gary Paul Nabhan, Wendy Hodgson, and Frances Fellows, "A Meager Living on Lava and Sand? Hia Ced O'odham Food Resources and Habitat Diversity in Oral and Documentary Histories," *Journal of the Southwest* 31 (December 1989), in press.

5. Miguel Velasco interview in Bell, Anderson, and Stewart, *Quitobaquito Cemetery*, p. 60.

6. Peter Raven, "Book Review: A Nostalgia for the Old Ways," *Natural History* (April-May 1989); Gary Paul Nabhan, *Enduring Seeds: Native American Agriculture and Wild Plant Conservation* (San Francisco: North Point Press, 1989).

7. Chona interview in Ruth Underhill, *Autobiography of a Papago Woman* (Menasha, Wis.: American Anthropological Assoc., 1936; reprint augmented ed., New York: Holt, Rinehart and Winston, 1979).

8. Venito García interview in Bell, Anderson, and Stewart, *Quitobaquito Cemetery*, p. 71.

9. For a discussion of outsiders' views of traditional O'odham Indian farming, see Nabhan, "Papago Indian Desert Agriculture," and Gary Paul Nabhan, "What Do You Do When the Rain Is Dying?" *The Desert Smells Like Rain: A Naturalist in Papago Indian Country* (San Francisco: North Point Press, 1982), p. 46.

10. Janette C. Brand, B. Janelle Snow, Gary P. Nabhan, and A. Stewart Truswell, "Plasma Glucose and Insulin Response to Traditional Pima Indian Meals," *American Journal of Clinical Nutrition* (1989), in press.

11. Compare the values in Brand, Snow, Nabhan, and Truswell, "Plasma Glucose and Insulin Response," with those in the extensive survey by D. J. A. Jenkins, T. M. S. Wolever, and R. M. Taylor, "Glycemic index of foods: a physiological basis for carbohydrate exchange," *American Journal of Clinical Nutrition* 36 (1981), pp. 362–66.

12. Brand, Snow, Nabhan, and Truswell, "Plasma Glucose and Insulin Response." See also A. C. Frati-Munari, B. E. Gordillo, P. Alamiro, and C. R. Ariza, "Hypoglycemic effect of *Opuntia streptacantha* Lemaire, in NIDDM," *Diabetes Care* 11 (1988), pp. 63–66; and Robert Becker, "Nutritive Value of Prosopis Pods," *Mesquite Utilization Symposium Proceedings* (Lubbock: Texas Tech University, 1982), p. M-1.

13. Boyd A. Swinburn and Vicki L. Boyce, "High-fat Diet Causes Deterioration in Glucose Tolerance, Insulin Secretion and Insulin Action," *Diabetes* (American Diabetes Association 49th Scientific Sessions) (May 1989).

14. Doris H. Calloway, R. D. Giaque, and F. M. Costa, "The Superior Mineral Content of Some American Indian Foods in Comparison to Federally Donated Counterpart Commodities," *Ecology of Food and Nutrition* 3 (1981), pp. 113–21.

15. Peter Alshire, "Experts Urge Diabetes Aid for Minorities," *Arizona Republic* 344 (Apr. 28, 1989); "A Su Salud" Hispanic Diabetes Conference agenda (American Diabetes Association, Arizona Affiliate, Inc., Phoenix).

16. Gary Paul Nabhan, "Replenishing Desert Agriculture with Native Plants and Their Symbionts," in Wes Jackson, Wendell Berry, and Bruce Colman, eds., *Meeting the Expectations of the Land: Essays in Sustainable Agriculture and Stewardship* (San Francisco: North Point Press, 1984), pp. 172–83.

17. Melvin R. Gilmore, "Uses of Plants by the Indians of the Missouri River Region," *Bureau of American Ethnology Annual Reports* 33 (1919), pp. 43–154.

18. Angelo Pellegrini, *The Unprejudiced Palate* (San Francisco: North Point Press, 1984), p. 229.

19. Nabhan, *Enduring Seeds,* p. 193.

20. Seventh Generation Fund, *Rebuilding Native American Communities* (Star Route, Lee, Nev.: Seventh Generation Fund Annual Report, 1987–1988), p. 16; Winona La Duke, "Native Rice, Native Hands: The Ikwe Marketing Collective," *Cultural Survival Quarterly* 2 (1987), pp. 63–65.

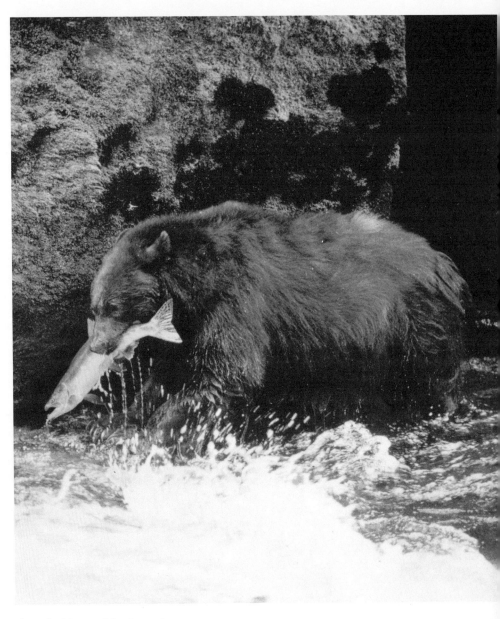

Photo by Tom and Pat Leeson.

The Last Columbia Salmon

Bruce Brown

The single-engined Cessna's stall buzzer shrieked like a teakettle as we executed a tight turn over the Wenatchee River at one thousand feet.

"Right, Willard, right," directed the state fisheries biologist from the copilot's seat. Willard, who was wearing a cowboy hat, nodded and rolled the plane over until his young companion literally hung over the scene he was studying so intently out the window.

The biologist, John Easterbrooks, followed the course of the river through a full body twist, stroked his beard, and jotted something in his notebook. Then, apparently satisfied with our second pass over a group of islands at the base of a red cliff, he directed Willard to continue upriver.

Instantly the throttle and flaps edged the kettle off the stove and reintroduced the sensations of weight and velocity. It was mid-October, and we were flying the Wenatchee River in search of wild chinook salmon, which can be spotted easily from the air by the yard-long nests they dig on the river bottom.

These nests, called redds, appear as light-colored ovals amid the darker, undisturbed gravel. It is here that Pacific salmon procreate and wait for the death that claims them all within a few days of mating. We had passed dozens of likely looking places on our flight up the river that morning, but we had seen no sign of salmon—just the empty river through neat apple orchards.

Our quarry was a particularly storied type of Pacific salmon. Popularly called chinook or king, they are the largest of the five species of Pacific salmon found in North America. The fish's Linnaean designation, *Oncorhynchus tshawytscha,* combines the

Latin for "hook nose" with the native Asian term for the fish. The most common North American name derives from the Chinook Indians, who controlled trade at the mouth of the Columbia River when Lewis and Clark arrived.

Two centuries ago, chinook ranged in Asia from the Japanese island of Hokkaido to the Anadyr River in Soviet Siberia. In North America, they were found from the Ventura River in Southern California near present-day Los Angeles to Point Hope, Alaska, well above the Arctic Circle, and possibly as far along the coast of the Arctic Ocean as Canada's Mackenzie River. On the Columbia, chinook ran in every month of the year, and they are still generally distinguished by the season they return to the river to spawn.

Spring chinook begin running into the rivers in May, headed for the glacier-fed headwater streams. Springers are the smallest of the chinook but also the richest, for they must live over half a year in fresh water on pelagic energy stored in their flesh. Summer chinook, which head for larger rivers in the deep canyon desert country, are the choicest commercially, since they combine rich flesh with greater size. Fall chinook are the least desirable, despite their weight. They run in from the ocean only a few weeks before they spawn, when their flesh is already wasted by approaching death, and spawn in the lower portions of the river.

Along the coasts of two continents, chinook and the other species of Pacific salmon used to feed virtually every predator imaginable from killer whales to grizzly bears, to bald eagles to water ouzels to humans. The fish were so numerous, in fact, that nothing could eat them all. Most of those returning from the sea succeeded in spawning. Then their rotting carcasses fed insects and plants that the next generation of juvenile salmon needed to survive.[1] In this way, the mass death of Pacific salmon—which at first seems so perverse a waste of procreative power—has actually been one of the keys to the fish's tremendous biological success.

We found our first salmon redds after about twenty minutes in the air. They were clustered right below U.S. 2 near the town of

Peshastin, the salmon acting out their rituals of mating and death a few feet from the thousands of motorists streaming by overhead. Heading upriver again, Easterbrooks said—yelled, actually—that the count of summer chinook in the lower Wenatchee that year was low. Ahead of us we could see the ersatz Tyrolean village of Leavenworth. If we were going to find wild summer chinook spawners in any numbers, it was probably going to be there, where the river emerges from Tumwater Canyon and the Cascade Mountains.

The Wenatchee River from the lower end of Tumwater Canyon to its confluence with Icicle Creek is the last mass summer chinook spawning ground remaining on the entire Columbia. There are scattered pockets of wild summer chinook spawning in other mid-Columbia tributaries, but the Leavenworth reach is the last place where you can still see wild summers take command of an entire section of river for their annual rites. "There it is," Easterbrooks said as we came in low and slow over a straight section of river about two hundred yards long. Willard had obviously flown this pattern before because he needed no directions as he rolled the plane across the face of the mountains and circled back around. Then he dropped the plane down between the tall cottonwoods on either side of the river so we could get a closer look.

Here where the mountain river enters the arid interior, the exceptionally clear water danced over a richly graveled bed. The river had thatched drift logs into the gravel, providing an unusual effect that was obviously very much to the salmon's liking. In some places, the logs cribbed up raised beds of clean gravel where the fish could dig their nests, while elsewhere the driftwood provided pikelike protection over deep holes where the fish could seek cover. Wild summer chinook had spawned all over the raised beds, so that it was impossible to tell where one redd ended and another began.

I did not see any salmon, though, until the second pass, when I realized the fish were not on their nests but rather in the deep green pools strewn along the river. Now I saw there were hundreds of salmon holding in loose schools that swayed with the current like sea grass. Occasionally, one or two of the gray-green fish broke away and seemed to chase their shadows through the logs. As I pressed against the cold, throbbing window of the plane, I thought of Lewis and Clark. In October 1805, near the confluence of the Snake and Columbia, they had observed tens of thousands of salmon flashing past in water "so clear that they could be seen down to a depth of 15 or 20 feet. The multitudes of this fish," they noted, "are almost inconceivable."

In those days, salmon was both the staple of the Columbia River Indians and the source of their choicest delicacies. The Indians of the Northwest Coast made a highly prized type of fermented "cheese" out of the caviar, while the natives of the Pacific Rim of Asia used salmon oil to fry a savory combination of sarana lily bulbs, marrow of purple fireweed, sweet grass, cloudberries, and crowberries.[2] Before the coming of the white man, North Pacific natives clothed themselves in brightly colored salmon-skin clothing, used the fish as a sort of currency, and even burned dried salmon for heat and illumination. Among commercial tribes like the Chinook, salmon also constituted the principal commodity of trade.

The influence of the salmon even extended to the spiritual realm. Most native people on the Pacific Rim of Asia and North America performed the first salmon ceremony at the beginning of the fishing season.[3] This ceremony ritually expressed the Indian belief that people and salmon are linked in a mirror world. The Kwakiutl Indians were one of the many tribes that believed that, beneath the ocean, salmon took the form of people and people took the form of salmon. They saw the salmon's annual migrations as a conscious sacrifice on their part for the benefit of mankind. The continuation of the runs was therefore in mankind's hands. If people did not act properly, the fish would not return.

The Indians called the largest salmon *tyee,* meaning "chief," and fished for them at cataracts, such as Kettle Falls, along the Columbia. Here, in 1860, Charles Wilson observed: "The falls are the most beautiful, the whole river falling over a ledge of quartz into a sort of cauldron in which the water bubbles and boils in the most remarkable fashion." Wilson, who was a

British member of the international commission that surveyed the western boundary between Canada and the United States, added that "the fishery, however, is the great sight and certainly is the most wonderful I ever saw. The salmon arrive at the foot of the falls in great numbers and proceed to leap them; all day long you see one continual stream of fish in the air."

The early whites called the choicest of the Columbia salmon bounty—the summer chinook—by another name. To them they were "June hogs," a term derived from the month of their spawning migration and their size—commonly in the seventy-five-pound range. Coming with the first good weather of the year, these prime summer chinook marked the climax of the early commercial fishery. In the glory days of the commercial Columbia fishery a century ago, forty million pounds of salmon—most of which was June hog—were shipped annually to the markets of the world from the Columbia in the form of canned salmon.

A picturesque river society of gill netters, pound netters, seiners, and trap operators grew up on the Columbia around the canneries. Rivalries among the various groups of white fishermen became so intense that they briefly provoked civil war between Oregon and Washington in 1887 when the Fisherman's Union struck for payment of one dollar per fish.[4] The mayhem and murder soon subsided, but the jostling for position among fishing groups continued until 1934 when small independent fishermen persuaded Washington to follow Oregon's example and outlaw mechanical salmon traps on the Columbia. Fishermen on the lower Columbia thought they had won a great victory for the salmon, but already a much greater threat to the Columbia chinook was taking shape.

In 1933, the federal government began building a 550-foot-high dam across the main-stem Columbia at Grand Coulee. "The mightiest thing ever built by a man," as Woody Guthrie sang, Grand Coulee Dam was intended to serve as a physical and symbolic cornerstone of President Franklin Roosevelt's New Deal. The idea was to harness the power of the Columbia—the largest North American tributary of the Pacific Ocean—to produce electrical power for jobs in the severely depressed Pacific Northwest, as well as to irrigate large tracts of fertile land for the benefit of the small farmers forced out of the Dust Bowl. Roosevelt also wanted to show Americans that, the Great Depression notwithstanding, they were still capable of great things.

The problem was that Roosevelt ordered a dam too high to pass fish over. This meant that all the salmon that spawned above Grand Coulee—roughly half the river's total salmon production—were exterminated when Grand Coulee closed its gates. The general public was never made aware of this fact, however. It is interesting to note that the original 1933 recommendation for Grand Coulee from the U.S. Army Corps of Engineers makes no mention of the fish that were the most conspicuous living feature of the Columbia basin. Nor was the loss of salmon calculated into the economic justification for what the corps' report acknowledged was a marginal irrigation project.[5]

Federal and state fisheries authorities raised some timorous protest over Grand Coulee, but they were silenced when the government promised to build three new salmon hatcheries in the mid-Columbia region on the Methow, Entiat, and Wenatchee rivers. There was no reason to believe that these salmon hatcheries could replicate the wild salmon runs killed by Grand Coulee, but the fisheries agencies' acceptance of the hatchery money gave the public the impression that the fishery would not be lost. It was a hopeful lie, and a crucial one to the symbolism of the big dam, for people might have looked differently on the enterprise if they had understood that it would destroy the region's richest source of free food at a time when people were actually starving.

By the end of World War II, the Grand Coulee compensation hatcheries had all failed and quietly been converted to other uses, such as raising trout. Thus the fabled June hogs of the Columbia vanished forever from the face of the earth. Their extermination made Grand Coulee Dam the single most destructive human act toward salmon in history, but it did not change public policy regarding dams and salmon on the Columbia.[6] Declaring that it now had the expertise to effect "the proper handling of the fish problem," the Army Corps of Engineers pressed for the construction of more than twenty new dams on the main-stem Columbia and Snake after World War II.

Most of these projects were built, and, like Grand Coulee, most included hatcheries that supposedly would "compensate" for the salmon they killed. Despite significant developments in the artificial propagation of salmon (such as the first disease-free feed, the Oregon moist pellet), not one of these hatcheries succeeded in replacing the wild salmon runs. The remaining Columbia River summer chinook run declined by another 50 percent between 1954 and 1977. There has not been a commercial summer chinook fishery on the Columbia since 1965, nor a tributary sports fishery since 1974. By 1978 all Columbia River salmon stocks were under consideration for inclusion on the federal government's threatened and endangered species lists.[7]

In some cases, hatchery salmon production, which continued to increase on the Columbia, actually helped speed the decline of the runs. An example is Wells Hatchery, which was built on the Columbia below Grand Coulee during the late 1960s to compensate for wild summer chinook spawning habitat destroyed by the Douglas County Public Utility District's Wells Dam. Unable, until recently, to return enough fish to spawn the next generation, the hatchery has been supported historically by draining the slight wild run that still ascends the fish ladders at Wells Dam. Year after year these summer chinook, which probably would survive better in the wilds, have been sacrificed to a barren hatchery. So the fish kill caused by the dam has been compounded by additional yearly losses at the hatchery (for which the public paid $500,000 during the first decade of operation alone).

Nor are the hatchery salmon physically identical to wild salmon of the same species. The most obvious difference is size. Hatchery salmon are generally smaller than their wild counterparts at maturity. The reason is the accelerated growth of hatchery fish. It turns out that speeding up the salmon's development in infancy (which is commonly done in hatcheries to save money) induces them to return from the ocean when they are younger and therefore smaller. In addition, some salmon connoisseurs, such as Dr. Charles Simenstad of the University of Washington's Fisheries Research Institute, claim they can taste the difference between wild and hatchery salmon "blindfolded, and maybe even in black bean sauce."

The most important difference between wild and hatchery salmon, though, may be their place in the ecology of the North Pacific Rim. In a region noted for its leaching rains, wild salmon serve as nature's main way of completing the cycle and returning nutrients from the ocean to the river. Hatchery salmon, by contrast, contribute little to the general ecosystem. Instead of feeding myriads, they are manipulated so that the majority of their benefit flows to just one species, humans, and only to the affluent few among us. Not too long ago, a fresh twenty-pound spring chinook sold for $120 in an Oregon supermarket.[8]

In 1982, a government report estimated that damming the Columbia had killed $6.5 billion worth of salmon over just the previous two decades. But dollars cannot begin to express the value of what has been lost. For millions of years, salmon and salmonlike creatures have been one of the central wellsprings around which life in the region has developed, matured, and maintained stability. With our dams, logging, farming, industrial pollution and such, we have virtually destroyed this vital system in the space of one century, and neither our electrical power nor our hatchery salmon can take its place.

"What do you think?" Easterbrooks asked as Willard pulled the plane up steeply and rolled to avoid the mountains directly ahead.

"That last time, I saw lots of fish," I said, gripping the seat in front of me. "There must be several hundred summer chinook holding together in the holes."

Willard brought us back around over the Leavenworth National Fish Hatchery on Icicle Creek, which was immediately recognizable by the large parking lot for tourists. Then we circled back to the Wenatchee, dropping down low once again and disturbing the concentration of the golfers on the eighteen-hole course that borders the river at the lower end of the summer chinook spawning glide.

Pulling out my camera, I counted off our last pass with what later proved to be strange, barely intelligible shots that made the salmon look like subatomic particles. Before I had finished a twenty-four-exposure roll, though, we had buzzed over the fish and come face to face once again with the mountains. This time, we rolled to the right toward the cliffs, heading for Tumwater Canyon.

I had an overpowering urge to tuck my arms against my sides as we entered the deep winding gorge, following the vein of jade-green water upriver toward a low dam. Although tiny compared to Grand Coulee, Tumwater Dam exterminated the salmon runs in the upper Wenatchee the same way that Grand Coulee had killed the June hogs: by blocking migration to their headwater spawning grounds.

Tumwater Dam would probably still block the Wenatchee today if not for the Pacific Northwest Power Planning Council. Created by Congress in 1980, the council is responsible for the overall planning and operation of the Pacific Northwest's massive hydroelectric power system. It has given the hydropower system its first unified leadership and the first regional power authority charged with considering factors other than electrical power. Not coincidentally, the council is the first Northwest power authority to emphasize the restoration of wild salmon runs.

On the main-stem Columbia and Snake rivers, the council forced the big dam operators to spill water for the sake of the fish, as well as to install devices to improve fish migration and reduce the dams' killing effect on the fish. On the Wenatchee River, it required the construction of fish passage facilities at Dryden and Tumwater dams. Similar work was performed on Oregon's Umatilla and Deschutes rivers. A great deal of habitat restoration work has also been carried out for the benefit of wild salmon on the Grande Ronde and John Day rivers, as well as several Idaho tributaries of the Snake.

"The council's clear preference for wild and natural stock propagation represents a significant departure from the recommendations of the fish and wildlife agencies, which considered artificial propagation to be 'the most critical element to assuring prompt recovery of spawning populations and the restoration of productive fisheries,' " said Michael Blumm of the Lewis and Clark Law School in Portland, Oregon. Blumm added that the fisheries agencies have been "particularly critical of the council's implication that the problems inherent in managing a mixed stock fishery [that is, a fishery composed of both hatchery and naturally spawned salmon] and the lack of harvest management controls [in the hands of the same fisheries agencies] were as culpable for the decline of the upriver runs as dam-caused habitat damage."

Even greater resistance to the Power Planning Council has come from the federal power agencies whose actions it is supposed to coordinate. In 1983, the Army Corps of Engineers refused to recognize orders from the council to spill water from its dams for salmon. And in 1984, the Bonneville Power Administration informed the council that it would pay for less than half the salmon restoration projects that the council had instructed it to carry out. The jurisdictional conflict came to a head that year when U.S. Senator Daniel Evans (a former chairman of the Power Planning Council) confronted emissaries from the power agencies face to face about their failure to comply with council directives.

Four months later, Evans successfully sponsored a bill in Congress to spend $30 million to make the Yakima River a pilot project for wild salmon restoration in the Columbia basin. Despite continued Corps of Engineers resistance on the Columbia and Snake, the council's Yakima salmon restoration project has installed fish ladders on more than a dozen irrigation diversion dams, among other improvements to increase salmon survival on the river. The council has also succeeded in forcing the laddering of dams on other Columbia tributaries, like Tumwater Dam on the Wenatchee.

The Yakima and the Wenatchee are still a long way from supporting a commercial chinook fishery again, but the early returns have been quite promising: Nearly ten thousand spring chinook ran into the Yakima in 1986. Now efforts are under way to reintroduce summer chinook on the Yakima, where they have been extinct for a quarter-century or more. The plan is to reseed the magnificent Yakima Canyon area with summer chinook from the Leavenworth stretch of the Wenatchee River.

Already the wild Wenatchee River summer chinook have

begun to reclaim their old spawning grounds in the vast upper Wenatchee above Tumwater Dam. We saw no fish above Tumwater Dam on our flight that day, but we did find something else that had been missing: hope. We knew that, despite the abuse heaped on the summer chinook of the Columbia, one vital ember remains.

I thought of the way the sun flashing on the Leavenworth salmon's backs made them look like a huge gem with countless living facets. The image stayed in my mind all the rest of the flight, which was so smooth we could have served tea.

Notes

1. For a ground-breaking scientific study of salmon carcass contribution to the riparian environment, see C. J. Cedarholm and N. P. Peterson, "The Retention of Coho Salmon Carcasses by Organic Debris in Small Streams," *Canadian Journal of Fisheries and Aquatic Sciences* (1985), pp. 1022–25.

2. A more extensive discussion of salmon in native cuisine is contained in Bruce Brown, *Mountain in the Clouds: A Search for the Wild Salmon* (New York: Touchstone, 1983), p. 23.

3. Much of the best material on the first salmon ceremony appeared in Erna Gunther, "An Analysis of the First Salmon Ceremony," *American Anthropologist* 28, no. 4 (October 1926), pp. 605–17 (first read before the British Association for the Advancement of Science in August 1924), and in her subsequent "A Further Analysis of the First Salmon Ceremony," *University of Washington Publications in Anthropology* 2, no. 5 (1928), pp. 129–72.

4. *Washington Salmon Fisheries on the Columbia River* (Vancouver, Wash.: Washington Fisheries Association, 1893), p. 3.

5. "Columbia River and Minor Tributaries: A Letter from the Secretary of War Transmitting . . . a Report, Together with Accompanying Papers and Illustrations, Containing a General Plan for the Improvement of the Columbia River and Minor Tributaries for the Purpose of Navigation and Efficient Development of Water-Power, the Control of Floods, and the Needs of Irrigation" (Washington, D.C.: Government Printing Office, 1933).

6. Anthony Netboy, *The Salmon: Their Fight For Survival* (Boston: Houghton-Mifflin, 1973) contains a good overview of mankind's long and destructive relationship with salmon in both the Pacific and Atlantic oceans.

7. *Summary of Workshop: Biological Basis for Listing Species or Other Taxa of Salmonids Pursuant to the Endangered Species Act of 1973* (Seattle: National Marine Fisheries Service, 1978).

8. A photo of a bemused supermarket manager holding the $120 fish in his arms appeared in the *Lake Oswego Review* and other Northwest publications in 1979.

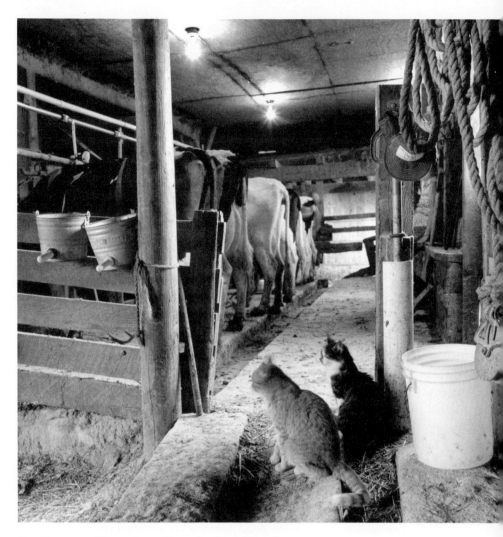

Cow Barn near Victor, Iowa. Photo by David Plowden.

Are Farmers an Endangered Species?

Mark Kramer

On a green weekend in midsummer, I visited five farmers, all at work within forty-five minutes of Boston Common, piloting energetic small businesses that work by commingling the special market circumstances of prosperous suburbia and the special personal circumstances that make their costly holdings of farm ground possible. Three run vegetable and flower farms (one has tried to remain organic). All have survived by using direct marketing, setting up farm stands, trucking to farmers' markets, arranging pick-it-yourself berry patches, and selling to the restaurants that take the trouble to order the freshest produce in town. All are run by young operators who have focused on the unique commercial ecology of plying a rural trade in suburbia. Some of them are what you'd expect—the lucky heirs of families that have farmed the same spots since land was cheap a few generations back. Jim Geoghegan, whose Sunshine Farm straddles the towns of Sherborn, Natick, and Framingham, says he feels fortunate that his siblings were farm-proud enough to join the business, preserving the home place.

What I *hadn't* expected to find was a new sort of farmer, like Tom Twomey of Highland Hill Farm, Holliston. After having worked for years for Stop and Shop as produce manager, he rallied his retired mother to run a farm stand and learned farming as his business grew. Another newcomer, Peter

Portions of this article come from the new Harvard University Press edition of *Three Farms: Making Milk, Meat, and Money from the American Soil.*

McArthur, liked his job in a greenhouse as a teenager and un-earthed a long farm lease from a conservation-minded land trust. He has poured himself into the tasks of building up green-houses and increasing his stand's business with the kind of glad, well-organized dedication that seems to define good farmers.

Bob Briggs runs one of the last independent dairies in Mas-sachusetts. Where land sells for $100,000 an acre, he tills a hundred acres, milking thirty holsteins and thirty jerseys, deliver-ing extrarich milk to five restaurants, and selling the rest—"in glass bottles because plastic and paper both leave a taste"—to townsfolk who drive to the farm and take it from a refrigerated case in the tiny bottling room off the barn. While I was there, some customers looked in on Briggs while he was milking. Others grabbed their milk and left their payment in a box. This may be the last place this side of the office coffee urn that dis-penses food on the honor system. In this special zone, 1954 rules still work well in 1989.

The fragile survival of this wonderful farm rests on the unexa-mined generosity of the burly Briggs, who simply says he keeps doing what he likes to do, which is the extraordinarily hard job of dairy farming. "My father began here in 1938," he relates. "He delivered his milk about town, as did others. He said he milked jerseys because, when you peddle house to house, you need an advantage, and taste was it. It still is. How many things in life can you look forward to? Even our skim milk tastes better, because jersey milk has higher milk-solids content as well as higher butterfat."

The final farmer I visited was in equally fragile circumstances. He's Jim Talvy, a brash young swashbuckler from suburbia, a modern man with a deft sense of business timing, a steady am-bition, a tolerance for large financial risk, and an atypical out-spokenness about the dairy industry's major issues. Talvy found a job on a dairy farm in Vermont one college summer, then married his boss's sister-in-law. He bought his own herd at the right moment—when the 1986 federal "whole-herd buyout" dropped cow prices for a few months. (The federal government that year bought and butchered 10 percent of our national dairy herd in order to lower surplus milk production.) Talvy rummaged about the world and found an anomalous landholding, a three-hundred-acre backwoods spread in otherwise suburbanized Upton, Massachusetts. The place had been farmed by a stubborn old Yankee who just wouldn't quit. In his frail final year, the old farmer rented his fields and barn to the young farmer, who had the sense to get a five-year lease. While the old man's heirs hash out the eventual division of the rolling land, the tax collector awaits payment of a huge estate tax.

Our hero has two more years to go in "Brigadoon" before it will be sold off for its "best and highest use," which, according to the shortsighted vote of the marketplace, is probably tract houses. By that time, Talvy will have a paid-for herd of registered holsteins, a full line of equipment, and the cash and cash flow to move on. The move will likely be out of state, to someplace far back where farmers still farm. "I'm not unhappy about it," he claims. "I'm lucky. I woke up at four-thirty this morning, and the day was beautiful. My cows are in great shape, and I had a good day from start to finish."

Yankee farming has become a delicate matter; it takes place in an atmosphere of siege. Its continuation is a matter of personal acts of sacrifice and goodwill. Nearly all farmers, until recently, have owned their farms, and anyone who bails out gets paid a million dollars by real estate developers — and ends up unemployed. Anyone who stays in it is quaint, a chump, a half-foolish hanger-on, cherished by neighbors who are glad of the open land and the wholesome local food production but who also wonder at the odd business judgment involved in electing hard work over wealth. The ones who farm on rented land farm for the foreseeable future, not for the ages.

In these modern times, in this prospering country, food is still love, and food is still culture, tradition, and pleasure, still the raw material of artfulness. But it is all these things only after the groceries leave the store and arrive home or reach a few, usually expensive, restaurants.

The bottom line counts more: We are all food addicts who must support our habit. Above all else, food is business. Our common hunger means money in someone else's bank account.

Our agriculture stayed quaint for a while longer than our steel mills did, but it has caught up. Today farming is big business. We grow food where it grows cheapest. We plant varieties, choose the species, material, methods, and labor that grow food cheapest. The outposts of quality I visited are self-conscious exceptions to the general trend. "I make some trade-offs," Tom Twomey, the former supermarket produce manager, told me. "We're growing for taste here at Highland Hill Farm, and we choose varieties accordingly. The gourmet is our market. They can get anything else everywhere else."

We lose small farmers. Farms grow bigger. A few of our farmers grow most of our food. Farming has become something distant from the lives of most Americans, something done not by one's grandparents, or cousins, or neighbors, but by assemblers of inputs — big businesses, located somewhere other than here, wherever "here" is, who pass on the material they produce for further processing elsewhere. With supermarkets full of food at reasonable cost, consumers forget other hungry nations' political instinct to cherish and guard their farmers. Our own dependence on ours slips out of mind. We abandon our awareness of biological and historical continuity, our knowledge of oneness with dirt and sun, our familiarity with the hand that feeds us.

In California and Iowa and Texas and Florida, while small farmers quit, the big ones persist — and buy up their failed neighbors. New England residents can also see the consolidation of farming. Here, where fields of over fifty acres are rare, when we lose small farmers we lose farming itself. America is on its way to being, boundary to boundary, a land of suburbanites, with farming and food handling handed over to the trust of a few large operators in every rural county, and with a few boutique minisuppliers for the urban carriage trade.

Quite naturally, most large farmers see their interests, with regard to industry's aggregate standards for chemical use, labor relations, quality, and marketing, as trade associations do. The stabilizing diversity that our food supply enjoyed when millions of farmers grew most of our food has disappeared. Some crops are already near-monopolies. Others, including some produce crops, are marketed in ways that create oligopolistic pricing conditions regionally and periodically. This system's triumph—the cheapness of food, which has driven and justified the system's transformation to date—may not last.

In my area, produce, nearly all of it imported from elsewhere even during the summer, costs 10 percent more than produce in other areas, and, of course, quality and selection suffer. Still, these days the supermarkets that give us our daily bread offer pretty and good-enough food in great array. The infrastructure of packers, shippers, and wholesalers that enables the miracle of supermarkets is as out of the public mind as farmers are. If this new concentration of food supply in the hands of an organized few were stable, then the new public unheedfulness might be tolerable. There are arguments—arguments of efficiency—for it. But the economy is not stable. It is always evolving, further perfecting itself, and we may lose more than the heritage we still remember; we may lose the efficient, healthy, quality food system that came to us because we started as a nation of farmers.

New England's near-farmlessness is an emblem—a blank emblem—of a national circumstance. Progress has seemed inexorable. It is an innocent process of a thousand subtle forces responding to opportunity, to freedom incarnate—a drama without villains. The large agricultural equipment now available operates most thriftily on large unbroken fields, but doesn't pay on hilly, small, widely separated Yankee fields. The coming of each technical innovation has hiked economies of scale—that is, the efficient size for a farm to be—further beyond the capacity of our terrain. The coming of milking parlors, automatic feeding, and high-production breeding not only through artificial insemination but also through ova transplantation has shifted efficient dairy herd size, for example, far above what a regional agriculture will support. Innocent progress has forced New England's milk supply to be grown out of the region and to be gathered and processed and resold by some of the food system's largest concerns.

You drive in the country here, and see a landscape-wide relic of the golden age of Yankee dairy farming just before the First World War, when an earlier round of technical advances began to take a toll on local farms. Just before tractors supplanted horses and milking machines replaced the farmer's hands, prospering farmers built farmhouse after farmhouse, each surrounded by ten cows' worth of land. Now, even mom-and-pop dairy farms can efficiently milk sixty to a hundred cows. So these days, mom and pop mostly live in Wisconsin. Most of their counterparts in Massachusetts have quit farming. The final slide is on here. We had a thousand dairies here three years ago. Now we have fewer than five hundred.

The few that survive are as amazing as they are rare. In every rural New England county, some farming families so clearly seem "elect" in their grace, good fortune, and optimistic outpouring of energy that their continuing constructive lives are worthy of celebration, as well as raised eyebrows. What is especially amazing about the five farmers I visited this summer is also true of the last four generations of some friends I have long admired, the Totman family of Conway, Massachusetts: They have made their farm thrive while New England agriculture on the whole has declined. Like horses so good they win races while carrying extra weight, they seem to improve under the strain of adversity. Their success at farming, especially in this hard place to farm, makes it easy to imagine how palpable that puritan notion of inborn elitism was to the citizens of Plymouth Plantation.

The elegance of these farmers' production is an elegance not of capital efficiency alone but of unalienated labor, of people justifiably engrossed in doing something worthwhile. This is the backdrop and setting that should remain at the heart of our consideration of food.

I meet Leland Totman one warm afternoon, as he maneuvers a silage wagon up to a silage blower. Chopped corn plants—ears, leaves, and stems alike, in spoon-sized bits—hurtle up sixty feet inside a tall stovepipe and topple down into the nearer of his two big round cement silos. It will ferment for two weeks, preserving itself, then will be fed out to cows all winter. "City people may not realize it," says Lee, "but hay isn't simply hay, and corn silage isn't simply corn silage."

This is as close as a real Yankee can come to boasting. Hay

can be stemmy, old, leafless, rained on, made from lackluster natural weed grasses. The hay in Lee's barn is always young, charcoal green, succulent, made from alfalfa, ladino clover, timothy grass, and red clover, containing 15 to 20 percent protein. Lee has hauled up corn fit for his regal cows, cut from fat corn plants that tasseled out higher than he can reach, bearing two long full ears of squat, deep kernels, plants the bright deep green of a child's crayon drawing of a corn plant, corn harvested in the prime of "hard dent" when the sugar content and nutrition are highest. The good corn and hay reflect Lee's attitude toward capital investment, toward how to succeed at farming where it's hard to farm; farming must make personal sense if he's to keep doing it, because he could sell out and be richer than he will be by staying.

I once saw Lee plowing under a stand of alfalfa and timothy that any other farmer in the county would have grown up and harvested proudly. "Didn't seem to be quite enough alfalfa in it," he said. When he got done plowing and disking and liming and fertilizing, he reseeded the field with the mixture he wanted there. When Lee's hay once got rained on badly, I saw him bale it up and give it away. "I'm not in the hay-selling business," he said. He sends his cull cows only to the butcher, never to other dairy farms. "I'm not in the breeding business," he says, "I'm in the milking business. I can't see saddling some other farmer with my problems."

When lesser farmers feel cramped for funds, the first place they cut is on field upkeep. A field in good shape is like stored money. The pressure on Lee is relentless. His land, put to use in the context of the harsh commercial structure of modern American dairying, teaches him the most compelling and relentless work ethic.

Just before milking time, we walk into the barn's great hall, the cows' "loafing shed," cool and smelling of corn and sawdust, manure and leather. It's spotless, whitewashed, scraped, newly bedded, empty. A long feed bunk runs up the center. Lee fills hayracks on the walls with his beautiful hay and throws a big switch at the base of the farthest silo. A motor whines, chains clank, belts slap into motion, and an automatic unloader delivers a stream of feed as it scoots along on a rail over the feed bunk.

The cows hear the noise and lumber up from pasture. His is a beautiful herd, a herd of Cadillacs, large, clean, coats shining, and with what cattle judges call "dairyness"—the undefinable look of an animal that means business—emanating from every beast. He watches them carefully for signs of heat, for health problems. We walk back through the loafing shed to the section of the barn called the milk house. We enter through a dark hallway, noisy with the roar of a compressor. The herd makes two thousand quarts a day.

Lee assembles three milking "claws." Their floppy juggling mouths of soft rubber will enfold the teats of each cow and draw milk from her in gentle wet pulses engineered to adore the udder in imitation of the mouth of a feeding calf. The milk will pass through the sterilized stainless steel tubing Lee is reassembling, clipping back into place. The milk moves from cow to truck without human touch.

He carries the assembled claws into the milking parlor. A waist-deep pit runs between cow stalls, three to a side. Cows assemble, walk in, are milked for six or seven minutes, walk out. The actual milking is Lee's payoff. It's routine. Everything that has gone before makes this part easy. The lead cows are in a hurry. The sound of sweet grain supplement falling into tin troughs sounds like hail on a tin roof. Three bushel-sized heads dunk into private luxury. Lee washes the cows' bags, their milk lets down; he plumbs them into the barn. The milk pulses from them with the sound of live calves suckling, the slow and imperious rhythm of living things, the steadying, hypnotic swish breathily repeating itself with the frequency of a healthy beating heart.

Milking time in Lee's parlor is as predictable as the counting of ballots in a Republican district. It's his time of solitude and repetitiveness, a meditation on a milky mantra, a compulsory, twice-daily trafficking with motherhood in its mammary, incarnadine quintessence. As the first three cows finish giving milk, he removes their machines and reattaches them to cows on the other side of the central pit, shoos the first three out, lets in three more to feed, get washed, and wait their turn. His is a laborious and tedious stewardship. He forgets himself, lost in the intricacies of the familiar chore.

The consuming nature of the profession makes our surviving dairy farmers a breed apart, who dwell amid a passage of events crucial to their survival but so intricate and private as to be incomprehensible to outsiders. Lee's vocation insulates him from the world. This may contribute to his decision to stay on when other farmers have abandoned Massachusetts consumers to drink milk from the thousand-cow farmerless factories farther west. His work is himself; he sticks to business. At the end of his sixteen-hour days, he falls asleep in front of the TV, and, as he tells me, he only dreams it's tomorrow, and he's out working again.

New technology offers as much threat to the surviving small dairy farmers of the nation as real estate brokers do. The harbingers of change aren't ones an outsider would see coming: One invention that has become standard on larger farms in the past decade automatically senses the cessation of milk flow, then removes the milking machines from the cows in the parlor, opens their stalls so they can return to pasture, opens the loafing shed door so three more cows can shoulder in, and lets grain rations fall into feeders for the new cows. This saves a farmer twenty seconds a cow—in other words, it *halves* the time spent milking each cow—and the freed time can be used to milk more cows. It's the sort of thing that makes farmers obsolete. Lee doesn't use this machine; he wants to watch his cows carefully so he'll spot health problems early.

Biotechnology is moving dairying in the same direction. Semen-sexing methods may soon allow cows to be bred to bear only female calves, doubling the dairy-calf selection from top cows. Ova transplants already allow average dairy mothers to host the fetuses of championship-quality calves. A barnful of drab moms can all drop world-class calves, doubling a herd's average production in a few years. And bovine growth hormone, a new bioengineered product that several chemical companies are now beginning to sell, promises to increase productivity in any cow by 10 to 15 percent. The product has not yet been sufficiently tested and seems to cause breeding difficulties, reduces the cows' end-of-lactation weight, and burns them out younger. Its effect on human health is unknown, and the impression it makes on consumers trained to appreciate the purity of milk is likely to be negative. It may come anyhow. It may not hurt people. Dairy cows die young anyway. Public perceptions can be adjusted. Americans don't stand long in the way of progress.

But all of these coming innovations will shrink the size of the national dairy herd, as fewer cows supply all the milk we need. This will make for ever larger dairy farms, run by ever fewer farmers. And the interests of a thousand-cow dairy factory in making thrifty milk will not be moderated by the interest Bob Briggs, Jim Talvy, and Lee Totman have in making milk that they are proud to offer their customers. If consumers who care pay attention to this link between small farmers and wholesome food, then they will know enough to try to hang on to what they value. In Massachusetts, for example, goaded by an extraordinary, activist commissioner of agriculture, the best restaurants and finest supermarkets in town have taken to promoting the fact that they buy locally grown food. Public sentiment has helped create the tax breaks that keep suburban farms in business and has enabled 265 farmers to place more than 25,000 acres of farmland in a state program that guarantees that it won't be developed in the future. The link between quality food and family farmers is worth recalling: It's us.

Growing Lean, Clean Beef

Gretel Ehrlich

In 1982, my husband and I bought a small mountain ranch in
northern Wyoming. An end-of-the-road place, arid, rough, and
beautiful, it had been badly neglected and abused. The house
was dark and dirty, the fences were in disrepair, no gates swung,
the outbuildings were roofless, the rangeland was badly overgrazed. But what an abundance of wildlife persists: Elk and deer
migrate through our hay fields in the spring and fall; shorebirds,
headed north, stop over on our big pond—avocets, terns,
godwits, phalaropes, rails, snipes, ducks, and even a whooping
crane. Mountain lions and black bear roam the steep canyons
and mountain slopes just above our house, golden and bald
eagles snatch up prairie dogs, ermine feed on baby cottontails,
cottontails snack on the vegetable garden I put in, a skunk bore
a litter of skunk kittens in a wild-rose thicket just outside my
study door.

In our restorative efforts, we have made the house livable,
rebuilt the sorting corrals, rewired miles of fence, and partially
rested our range. When we bought our own cattle, our idea was
to raise lean, clean beef in an environmentally sound way. This
brought derisive smiles to many faces. The unsound agricultural
practices of farmers and ranchers have contributed to an estimated 50 percent of the deterioration of the planet's natural
resources. It's an old story: the dumping of chemicals onto
the ground and into animals; overgrazing and the desertifica-
tion of the planet; the use of disease-ridden feedlots and
the subsequent emission of methane into the atmosphere—

all of which adds up to raising unhealthy food in a destructive, ecologically unhealthy way.

The ironic inconsistencies are bewildering. Food has to do with love. It is one of the means by which the human learns self-transcendence. Our bodies are capable of making food as well as of ingesting it or, as with Jonah, of being ingested by another animal. Being fed is the first cultural act we experience in our lives; growing and eating food constitutes our primordial connection to the planet for, through our dual role as nurturer and predator, we forge our citizenship in the natural world.

Masanobu Fukuoka, who practices a Taoist-style "do-nothing," natural way of farming, wrote in his book *The One-Straw Revolution:* "People eat with their minds, not their bodies. . . . When people rejected natural food and took up refined food instead, society set out on a path toward its own destruction. This is because such food is not the product of true culture. Food is life, and life must *not* step away from nature."

Agriculture has turned into a culture of death. Farmers and ranchers go bankrupt; we lose six tons of topsoil for every ton of grain produced; thirty calories of fossil energy are spent for each calorie of food eaten; our aquifers are being drained; our ranges have been overgrazed for a hundred years. Areas of the United States are desertifying as quickly as places in Africa. Environmentalists fight ranchers who fight federal agencies that manage public land and handle every so-called natural disaster, many of which, like drought, are caused by humans and are met with crisis-oriented Band-Aid solutions that perpetuate the problem in the long run. People would rather complain than collaborate, because accepting new ideas, working together, and putting long-term solutions into practice requires discipline within a culture that stimulates only undisciplined, insatiable need and greed. But it is pointless to lay blame; it makes sense only to find and practice solutions. And every problem, though local, must be solved with a global eye.

Our early efforts at recovering the range that goes with our ranch, as well as at restoring watersheds, were semifailures. We reduced the stocking rate of cattle by half (numbers of animals per acre per month), put them on the range late and took them off early, but this "partial rest" improved the grass only slightly. With an increasingly severe drought (still going on at this writing), the water situation became critical. Our riparian areas had been denuded of vegetation, and nothing we were doing was helping to hold the moisture in the ground. We were, of course, looking at the wrong things in the wrong way.

In 1987, my husband and I enrolled in courses at the Center for Holistic Resource Management based in Albuquerque, New Mexico, and founded by Allan Savory, whose breakthrough ideas have created new guidelines for using old management tools. Almost three thousand people, including ranchers, hired hands, Bureau of Land Management and Forest Service personnel, wildlifers, conservationists, and environmentalists, have taken courses offered by the center, enabling many of us to rethink ourselves, our finances, and our ecosystems.

Holistic resource management isn't an agricultural system; it's a thought process, an acknowledgment of a natural world functioning in wholes that are composed of lesser wholes. Any management ideas that don't consider the entire ecosystem risk destroying that ecosystem. The process by which one can manage a ranch, a national park, a farm, or anything else, for that matter, is by setting goals that include the quality of life, the landscape, and the production desired. Only after these are set should we consider the vast array of means by which to achieve these goals and then test the means against cultural, financial, and biological guidelines. The key, Allan Savory says, is understanding that natural resources are part of a whole, so no single goal or problem can be dealt with independently of its effect on the whole.

After these courses, I began going for long walks. From a high mountain slope above the ranch, I looked down on the hundred-year-old house, the sorting corrals hacked from cedar and fir with a hand ax. I got down on my hands and knees on the range, in the hay meadows. What is growing, how fast, when, why, where? How have humans changed the landscape, how will it look a hundred years from now? What is a ranch? What are the actual ingredients with which I am working? I answered the

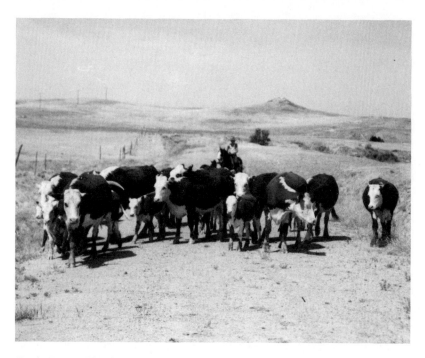

Cattle Drive, Glendive, Montana, July 1936. Photo by Arnold Rothstein.

last two questions first, and they changed the way I looked at all the others. A ranch is soils, plants, humans, animals. The ingredients with which I work are minerals, water cycles, and sunlight. A ranch is a cultural site mostly made of sun. I'm not producing lean beef, I'm ranching sunlight, and, in managing for successional complexity—that is, for more grass, less bare soil surface, more insects, birds, and mammals—I'm encouraging the conversion of sunlight into other forms of energy: food for livestock; food for humans; and what Allan Savory calls "solar dollars," or nature's gifts, which sometimes take the form of currency, sometimes the form of more cows and calves, streams that flow year-round, or the end of a drought and the beginning of rainy seasons.

A rancher's year can be said to begin in midwinter, when the calves start to come. My journal entries for February and March all read 1:00 A.M., 2:45 A.M., 3:00 A.M., because that's when I get up to check first-calf heifers and "calvy" cows. Trudging through snow, I turn my flashlight on the contours of their heaving bodies. When a cow's water breaks or I see feet emerging, I stay with her and help with the birth if necessary. During the day, I doctor sick calves, bottle-feed a bum calf, lay out straw under protective trees for the night because the cold here is often deeper than the snow.

By the end of March, I feel so deeply connected to these animals' lives that I forget we are a different species. Sleeplessness and the adrenaline of the calving barn push me into an indisputable sense of equality: My existence is as accidental and precarious as any calf's. Under the smoke-colored limbs of willow trees, the cows' collective breath — with mine added — forms a cloud of mist that vanishes the way a thought does. My husband and I develop a bovine, maternal ESP: One of us will suddenly jump up and go to the calving pasture, knowing our help is needed or that something has gone wrong.

In May we turn the cows and calves out onto the range. It is now known that overgrazing is a function of time rather than numbers of animals. In other words, if one cow, horse, or ewe is left long enough on a thousand-acre pasture, that chunk of land will be as overgrazed as it would be if a thousand animals had been put on it. Given enough time, a grazing animal will go back to the most palatable plant over and over, thus weakening the root system and the plant's ability to trap sunlight with its green-leaf surface.

The western states have been overgrazed since the 1880s (earlier in California and New Mexico where the Spaniards dumped thousands of animals on the land). The natural productive capacity of the land was enormous before domestic livestock was introduced, even though the grass was being grazed by buffalo. Because one of our goals is to manage for species diversity as well as for the production of chemical-free, naturally lean beef, we decided to use cattle as a tool for restoring the health of the range and at the same time get the dividends from the sale of our beef.

The key lies in simulating the grazing patterns of the buffalo and the predator-prey relationships that formed those patterns. We use, in lieu of predators (no wolves—yet—and no humans with obsidian spears), a single strand of electric fence wire, lightweight portable posts, and solar energizers for time-controlled grazing.

Out of large pastures, we create relatively small ones in which cattle are allowed to graze for a number of days (say, three to five) determined by the rate of plant growth and the numbers of acres and animals. When the time is up, they are moved to the next enclosure so that, ideally, no grass plant is grazed more than once. On our ranch, these small, temporary pastures are not grazed again for an entire year.

Thus, riparian (streamside) areas are never grazed for more than a few days, which prevents cattle from using these fragile places as a private lounge. We do transects, monitoring numbers of species, distance between grass plants, evidence of animal life in the area, and quality of the soil surface. A healthy ecosystem has porous soil with a natural mulch of litter, new seedlings in among mature grass plants, and a healthy level of succession indicated by the presence of ants, worms, bees, birds, rabbits, deer, elk, and so on. We plan, monitor, and replan because any ecosystem is a dynamic, changing thing; if we lose our flexibility, we will fail to stay contemporary with the changes in the air and on the ground.

In October, when most Wyoming ranchers sell their calves to feedlots, we wean and keep our steer calves over for another year. We know that feedlots are disease-ridden, that the cattle are fed grain and corn laced with antibiotics, and that no animal taken off any high mountain pasture in Wyoming could be happy in such a place. Our steers are ranch-raised and grass-fed. Twenty days before butchering, they receive local, organically grown grain as a supplement to their diet of high-protein, high-altitude grass and home-grown grass and alfalfa hay. Just about the time the wild ducks that use our pond all summer have grown flight feathers, our eighteen-month-old steers go to the processor. The meat is cut, wrapped, and flash frozen, then shipped by overnight air to the consumer.

Soon enough winter comes. We use wood heat and cook on

an old stove. It's the time of year when we rethink our biological and land planning and add up our profits and losses. When the snow gets too deep, we feed our cattle and horses using a team of Belgian horses. (Horses aren't hard to start when it's 30° below.) The last five years of drought have taken their toll on our place, yet we've still had successes. Grasses have increased from five to twenty native perennial species. The resident herd of elk has increased by fifteen head. Springs have begun running where none existed before; we protect them at the source and develop the water. And this year we might even make some money.

When we manage for plenty, for what Gary Snyder calls "the good, wild, and sacred," an internal sense of fullness arises. Once we understand where and why life occurs and how to stop destroying it, a mindfulness about everything spreads. The land tells us what it needs and when; we just have to be awake, to listen, and to scrutinize the ground. Now, every time I go for my walk, I see more—and the more I see, the more I see. Abundance is contagious. That's how life on the earth came to be, how plants and animals coevolved, each unique detail profoundly connected to the whole. I laughingly refer to our ranch as "my laboratory"—only it's nature who does her experiments on me, not the other way around. No day goes by when I'm not bowled over by something—the way the ravens play hide-and-seek in the trees; the way the spring sky is lit simultaneously by the aurora in the north and lightning in the south; the way my working dogs and horses anticipate what I'm thinking of doing next through the subtle, complex cues they use to know me; and, in late June, the way the elk bring their calves down to the benchland east of our house as if to show us their young, which were conceived in a chaos of rut in the field just below.

A ranch is a teacher. When we move in the direction of the land's health, from the ground up, the health of the animals we raise—sired by salers bulls, out of red angus cows—is ensured.

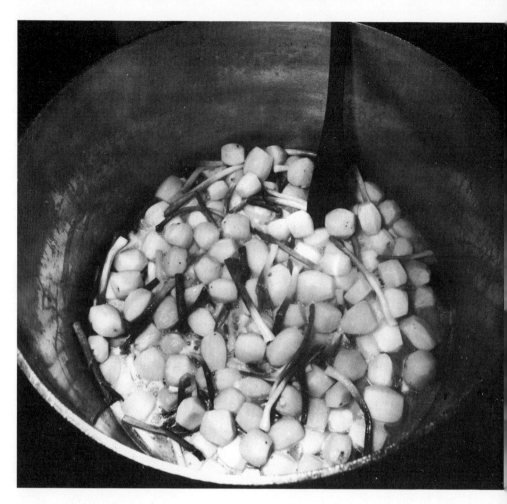

Photo by Gail Skoff.

The Farm–Restaurant Connection

Alice Waters

I have always believed that a restaurant can be no better than the ingredients it has to work with. As much as by any other factor, Chez Panisse has been defined by the search for ingredients. That search and what we have found along the way have shaped what we cook and ultimately who we are. The search has made us become part of a community—a community that has grown from markets, gardens, and suppliers and has gradually come to include farmers, ranchers, and fishermen. It has also made us realize that, as a restaurant, we are utterly dependent on the health of the land, the sea, and the planet as a whole, and that this search for good ingredients is pointless without a healthy agriculture and a healthy environment.

We served our first meal at Chez Panisse on August 28, 1971. The menu was pâté en croûte, duck with olives, salad, and fresh fruit, and the meal was cooked by Victoria Wise, who, together with Leslie Land and Paul Aratow, was one of the three original cooks at the restaurant. The ducks came from Chinatown in San Francisco and the other ingredients mostly from two local super-markets: the Japanese produce concession at U-Save on Grove Street and the Co-op across the street. We sifted through every leaf of romaine, using perhaps 20 percent of each head and dis-carding the rest. We argued about which olives we ought to use with the duck and settled without much enthusiasm on green ones whose source I don't recall, agreeing after the fact that we could have done better. To this day we have yet to find a source of locally produced olives that really satisfies us.

We don't shop at supermarkets anymore, but in most respects the same processes and problems apply. Leslie Land recalls, "We were home cooks—we didn't know there were specialized restaurant suppliers. We thought everybody bought their food the way we did." I think that ignorance was an important, if unwitting, factor in allowing Chez Panisse to become what it is. Often, we simply couldn't cook what we wanted to cook because we couldn't find the level of quality we needed in the required ingredients, or we couldn't find the ingredients at all. Our set menus, which we've always published in advance so customers can choose when they want to come, featured the phrase "if available" with regularity during the first seven or eight years. Since we've always felt that freshness and purity were synonymous with quality, there were few guarantees that what we needed would appear in the form and condition we wanted when we wanted it.

If, as I believe, restaurants are communities—each with its own culture—then Chez Panisse began as a hunter-gatherer culture and, to a lesser extent, still is. Not only did we prowl the supermarkets, the stores and stalls of Chinatown, and such specialty shops as Berkeley then possessed (some of which, like the Cheese Board and Monterey Market, predated us and continue to develop from strength to strength) but we also literally foraged. We gathered watercress from streams, picked nasturtiums and fennel from roadsides, and gathered blackberries from the Santa Fe tracks in Berkeley. We also took herbs like oregano and thyme from the gardens of friends. One of these friends, Wendy Ruebman, asked if we'd like sorrel from her garden, setting in motion an informal but regular system of obtaining produce from her and other local gardeners. We also relied on friends with rural connections: Mary Isaak, the mother of one of our cooks, planted fraises des bois for us in Petaluma, and Lindsey Shere, one of my partners and our head pastry cook to this day, got her father to grow fruit for us near his place in Healdsburg.

Although most of our sources in the restaurant's early days

were of necessity unpredictable, produce was the main problem area, and we focused our efforts again and again on resolving it. Perhaps more than any other kind of foodstuff, produce in general and its flavor in particular have suffered under postwar American agriculture. Although we've been able to have as much cosmetically perfect, out-of-season fruit and vegetables as anyone could possibly want, the flavor, freshness, variety, and wholesomeness of produce have been terribly diminished. With the notable exception of Chinese and Japanese markets that even in the early seventies emphasized flavor and quality, we really had nowhere to turn but to sympathetic gardeners who either already grew what we needed or would undertake to grow it for us.

Our emphasis—and, today, our insistence—on organically grown produce developed less out of any ideological commitment than out of the fact that this was the way almost everyone we knew gardened. We have never been interested in being a health or natural foods restaurant; rather, organic and naturally raised ingredients happen to be consistent with both what we want for our kitchen and what we want for our community and our larger environment. Such ingredients have never been an end in themselves, but they are a part of the way of life that inspired the restaurant and that we want the restaurant to inspire. Most of us have become so inured to the dogmas and self-justifications of agribusiness that we forget that, until 1940, most produce was, for all intents and purposes, organic, and, until the advent of the refrigerated boxcar, it was also of necessity fresh, seasonal, and local. There's nothing radical about organic produce: It's a return to traditional values of the most fundamental kind.

It had always seemed to us that the best way to solve our supply problems was either to deal directly with producers or, better still, to raise our own. By 1975, we'd made some progress with the first approach, regularly receiving, for example, fresh and smoked trout from Garrapata in Big Sur. One of my partners, Jerry Budrick, had also set up a connection with the Dal Porto Ranch in Amador County in the foothills of the Sierra Nevada, which provided us with lambs and with zinfandel grapes for the house wine Walter Schug made for us at the

Joseph Phelps Winery. Jerry also acquired some land of his own in Amador, and it seemed an obvious solution to our produce needs for us to farm it. In 1977 we tried this, but we knew even less about farming than we thought we did, and the experiment proved a failure.

Fortunately, during the late 1970s some of our urban gardens were producing quite successfully, notably one cultivated by the French gardener and cook at Chez Panisse, Jean-Pierre Moullé, on land in the Berkeley hills owned by Duke McGillis, our house doctor, and his wife, Joyce. In addition, Lindsey Shere returned from a trip to Italy laden with seeds, which her father planted in Healdsburg, thereby introducing us to rocket and other greens still exotic at that time. Meanwhile, we were also learning how to use conventional sources as best we could. Mark Miller, then a cook with us, made the rounds of the Oakland Produce Market each dawn, and we discovered useful sources at other wholesale and commercial markets in San Francisco. Closer to home, we bought regularly—as we still do—from Bill Fujimoto, who had taken over Monterey Market from his parents and had begun to build its reputation for quality and variety.

It's difficult now to remember the kind of attitude to flavor and quality that still prevailed in the mid and late 1970s. When Jeremiah Tower, who was our main cook at Chez Panisse from 1973 to 1977, once sent back some meat he felt wasn't up to scratch, the supplier was apoplectic: No one had ever done that before. And Jerry Rosenfield, a friend and physician who has worked on many of our supply problems over the years, caused an uproar one morning when he was substituting for Mark Miller at the Oakland Produce Market: Jerry insisted on *tasting* some strawberries before buying them. Jerry was also a key figure in securing our sources for fish, probably the first of our supply problems that we were able to solve successfully. During the restaurant's first few years, we served very little fish at all, such was the quality available—despite our being across the bay from a city renowned for its seafood. But, in 1975, Jerry brought us some California sea mussels he'd gathered near his home, and they were a revelation. We asked him to bring us more, and in late 1976 he became our fish dealer, buying from wholesalers and fishermen ranging up the coast from Monterey to Fort Bragg. Along the way he began to be assisted by Paul Johnson, a cook from another Berkeley restaurant called In Season, who took over from Jerry in 1979 and who today sells what is arguably the best fish on the West Coast.

Our produce problem, however, remained unsolved, and we decided to have another try at farming. John Hudspeth, a disciple of James Beard who later started Bridge Creek restaurant just up the street from us, owned some land near Sacramento that he was willing to make available to us in 1980 and 1981. In some respects, this farm was a success—producing good onions and potatoes and wonderful little white peaches from a tree John had planted—but we weren't equipped to deal with the valley heat or the land's penchant for flooding. While the farm did produce, it produced unreliably, and we had to continue to obtain supplies from elsewhere. It also finally disabused us of any illusion that we were farmers. We realized that there seemed to be only two solutions available: extending and formalizing the system of urban gardeners we already had in place, and establishing direct connections with sympathetic farmers who could grow what we needed—that is, farmers who, since we didn't know enough farming to do it ourselves, would farm on our behalf.

In the early 1980s, two members of the restaurant staff, Andrea Crawford and Sibella Kraus, and Lindsey Shere's daughter Thérèse established several salad gardens in Berkeley, one of which was in my backyard. These eventually met most of our needs for salad greens, but for other kinds of produce we remained dependent on a hodgepodge of often-unreliable sources. Two things happened in 1982, however, that turned out to be tremendously important. First, Jean-Pierre Gorin, a friend and filmmaker teaching in La Jolla, introduced us to the produce grown near there by the Chino family. And, second, Sibella Kraus became the forager for the restaurant and eventually started the Farm-Restaurant Project. Jean-Pierre happened by the Chinos' roadside stand, tasted a green bean, and arranged to have two boxes sent to us immediately. The beans were exquisite, and I flew down to find out who had grown them. We became good friends, and to this day we receive nine boxes of produce from the Chinos each week.

Meanwhile, as Sibella had become more and more involved with our salad gardens, she decided that she would like to work with produce full-time and proposed that she become the restaurant's first full-time forager, an idea we agreed to with enthusiasm. Sibella spent her time on the road locating farmers, tasting their produce, and, if we liked it, arranging for a schedule of deliveries to Chez Panisse. In 1983, we funded the Farm-Restaurant Project under Sibella's direction, which set up a produce network among a number of Bay Area restaurants and local farmers and culminated in the first Tasting of Summer Produce, now an annual event at which dozens of small, quality-conscious farmers show their produce to the food community and the general public. Sibella left us to work for Greenleaf Produce (from whom we still regularly buy) and has become an important figure in the sustainable-agriculture movement. She was succeeded as forager by Catherine Brandel, who has since become one of the head cooks in our upstairs café. During this period, Green Gulch, run by the San Francisco Zen Center, became an important supplier, as did Warren Weber, whom we continue to work with today. We were also fortunate to have Thérèse Shere and Eric Monrad producing tomatoes, peppers, beans, lettuce, and lamb for us at Coulee Ranch near Healdsburg.

During her tenure as forager, Catherine continued to develop the network Sibella had created, finding, for example, a regular source of eggs for us at New Life Farms. But she was frustrated, as we all were, by the seeming impossibility of finding meat that was both flavorful and raised in a humane and wholesome way. Since the beginning of Chez Panisse, we had been forced to rely on conventional suppliers, a continuing disappointment given how much progress we had made with other kinds of materials. But, in late 1986, Jerry Rosenfield took over as forager from Catherine, and over the next two years he made enormous strides in finding meat sources for us. Jerry had been living in the Pacific Northwest and had discovered a number of ranchers and farmers there who were attempting to raise beef, veal, and lamb without hormones and under humane conditions. In particular, the Willamette Valley between Portland and Eugene, Oregon, became a source for rabbits, lambs, goats, and beef, although Jerry also located producers closer to home, including ones for game and for that most elusive bird—a decently flavored, naturally raised chicken. We still have a way to go, but today, for the first time in our history, we are able to serve meat that really pleases us.

We have made progress on other fronts, too. In 1983, for example, we helped Steve Sullivan launch Acme Bakery, which bakes for us and for many other local restaurants. And, recently, we've realized a close approximation of our dream of having a farm. In 1985, my father, Pat Waters, began looking for a farmer who would be willing to make a long-term agreement to grow most of our produce for us according to our specifications. With help from the University of California at Davis and local organic food organizations, Dad came up with a list of eighteen potential farmers, which he narrowed down to a list of four on the basis of interviews, tastings, and visits. We settled on Bob Cannard, who farms on twenty-five acres in the Sonoma Valley.

Bob is very special, not only because he grows wonderful fruits and vegetables for us—potatoes, onions, salad greens, tomatoes, beans, berries, peaches, apricots, and avocados, to name a few—but also because he is as interested in us as we are in him. He likes to visit the restaurant kitchen and pitch in, and we send our cooks up to him to help pick. He takes all the restaurant's compostable garbage each day, which he then uses to grow more food. He is also a teacher at his local college and a major force in his local farmer's market. He sees that his farm and our restaurant are part of something larger and that, whether we acknowledge it or not, they have a responsibility to the health of the communities in which they exist and of the land on which they depend.

The search for materials continues, and I imagine it always will. We are still looking for good sources for butter, olives, oil, and prosciutto, to name a few. But, even when we find them, the foraging will continue. Ingredients will appear that we'll want to try, and we in turn will have new requirements that we'll want someone to fulfill for us. Whatever happens, we realize that, as restaurateurs, we are now involved in agriculture and its vagaries—the weather, the soil, and the economics of farming and rural communities. Bob Cannard reminds us frequently that farming isn't manufacturing: It is a continuing relationship with nature that has to be complete on both sides to work. People claim to know that plants are living things, but the system of food production, distribution, and consumption we have known in this country for the last forty years has attempted to deny that they are. If our food has lacked flavor—if, in aesthetic terms, it has been dead—that may be because it was treated as dead even while it was being grown. And perhaps we have tolerated such food—and the way its production has affected our society and environment—because our senses, our hearts, and our minds have been in some sense deadened, too.

I've always felt it was part of my job as a cook and restaurateur to try to wake people up to these things, to challenge them really to taste the food and to experience the kind of community that can happen in the kitchen and at the table. Those of us who work with food suffer from an image of being involved in an elite, frivolous pastime that has little relation to anything important or meaningful. But in fact we are in a position to cause people to make important connections between what they are eating and a host of crucial environmental, social, and health issues. Food is at the center of these issues.

This isn't a matter of idealism or altruism but rather one of self-interest and survival. Restaurateurs have a very real stake in the health of the planet, in the source of the foodstuffs we depend on, and in the future of farmers, fishermen, and other producers. Hydroponic vegetables or fish raised in pens will never be a real substitute for the flavor and quality of the ingredients that are in increasing jeopardy today. Professionally and personally, both our livelihoods and our lives depend on the preservation of what we have and the restoration of what we have lost. The fate of farmers—and with them the fate of the earth itself—is not somebody else's problem: It is our fate, too.

There is clearly so much more to do. But ultimately it comes down to realizing the necessity of the land to what we do and our connection to it. Few restaurants are going to be able to create the kind of relationship we have with Bob Cannard, but there are other routes to the same goal. I'm convinced that farmer's markets are an important step in this direction; they also contribute to the local economy, promote more variety and quality in the marketplace, and create community. As restaurateurs and ordinary consumers meet the people who grow their food, they acquire an interest in the future of farms, of rural communities, and of the environment. This interest, when it helps to ensure the continuing provision of open space near cities and the diversity of food produced on it, is to everyone's benefit. Country and city can once again become a mutual support system, a web of interdependent communities. That's why fresh, locally grown, seasonal foodstuffs are more than an attractive fashion or a quaint, romantic notion: They are a fundamental part of a sustainable economy and agriculture—and they taste better, too. Of course, people respond, "That's easy for you to say: In California you can have whatever you want all year round." I tell them that's true, but I also tell them that most of it tastes terrible. And, while there's no reason to forgo all non-locally-produced ingredients—I wouldn't want to give up our weekly shipment from the Chinos—local materials must become the basis of our cooking and our food; this is true for every region of the planet that has produced a flavorful, healthy cuisine.

What sometimes seem to be limitations are often opportunities. Earlier this year, in the lee between the early spring vegetables and those of mid-summer, we had an abundance of fava beans, which we explored in the kitchen for six weeks, served in soups, in purees, as a garnish, and, of course, by themselves— and we discovered that we had only *begun* to tap the possibilities. There was a stew of beans with savory and cream, a fava-bean-and-potato gratin, fava bean pizza with lots of garlic, a pasta fagioli using favas, a rough puree of favas with garlic and sage, and a vinaigrette salad, to name a few. The point is that what constitutes an exciting, exotic ingredient is very much in the eye of the beholder and that few things can be as compelling as fresh, locally grown materials that you know have been raised in a responsible way.

When I was first thinking about opening what would become Chez Panisse, my friend Tom Luddy took me to see a Marcel Pagnol retrospective at the old Surf Theater in San Francisco. We went every night and saw about half the movies Pagnol made during his long career, including *The Baker's Wife* and his Marseilles trilogy—*Marius, Fanny,* and *César.* Every one of these movies about life in the south of France fifty years ago radiated wit, love for people, and respect for the earth. Every movie made me cry.

My partners and I decided to name our new restaurant after the widower Panisse, a compassionate, placid, and slightly ridiculous marine outfitter in the Marseilles trilogy, so as to evoke the sunny good feelings of another world that contained so much that was incomplete or missing in our own—the simple wholesome good food of Provence, the atmosphere of tolerant camaraderie and great lifelong friendships, and a respect both for the old folks and their pleasures and for the young and their passions. Four years later, when our partnership incorporated itself, we immodestly took the name Pagnol et Cie., Inc., to reaffirm our desire to recreate a reality where life and work were inseparable and the daily pace left time for the afternoon anisette or the restorative game of *pétanque,* and where eating together nourished the spirit as well as the body—since the food was raised, harvested, hunted, fished, and gathered by people sustaining and sustained by each other and by the earth itself. In this respect, as in so many others, the producers and farmers we have come to know not only have provided us with good food but have also been essential in helping us to realize our dreams.

THREE

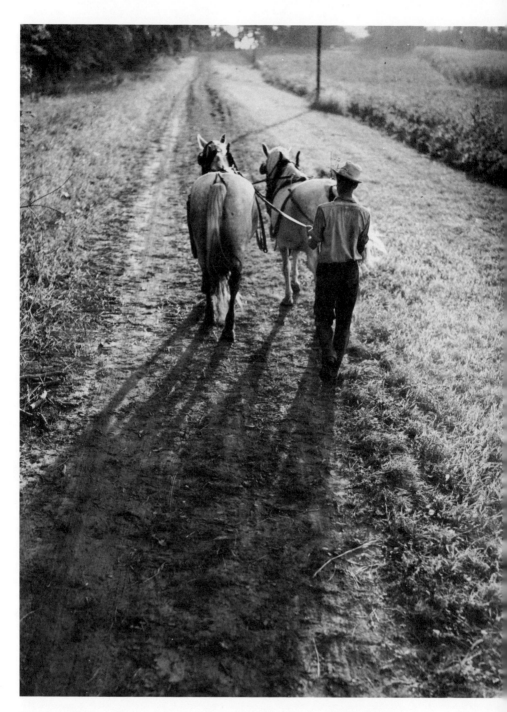

Farmer and Team, Hardin County, Iowa, 1939. Photo by Arnold Rothstein.

The Pleasures of Eating
Wendell Berry

Many times, after I have finished a lecture on the decline of American farming and rural life, someone in the audience has asked, "What can city people do?"

"Eat responsibly," I have usually answered. Of course, I have tried to explain what I meant, but afterwards I have invariably felt that there was more to be said than I had been able to say. Now I would like to attempt a better explanation.

I begin with the proposition that eating is an agricultural act. Eating ends the annual drama of the food economy that begins with planting and birth. Most eaters, however, are no longer aware that this is true. They think of food as an agricultural product, perhaps, but they do not think of themselves as participants in agriculture. They think of themselves as "consumers." If they think beyond that, they recognize that they are passive consumers. They buy what they want—or what they have been persuaded to want—within the limits of what they can get. They pay, mostly without protest, what they are charged. And they mostly ignore certain critical questions about the quality and the cost of what they are sold: How fresh is it? How pure or clean is it, how free of dangerous chemicals? How far was it transported, and what did transportation add to the cost? How much did manufacturing or packaging or advertising add to the cost? When the food product has been "manufactured" or "processed" or "precooked," how has that affected its quality or nutritional value?

Most urban shoppers would tell you that food is produced on farms. But most of them do not know on what farms, or what kinds of farms, or where the farms are, or what knowledge or skills are involved in farming. They apparently have little doubt that farms will continue to produce, but they do not know how or over what obstacles. For them, then, food is pretty much an abstract idea—something they do not know or imagine—until it appears on the grocery shelf or on the table.

The specialization of production induces specialization of consumption. Patrons of the entertainment industry, for example, entertain themselves less and less and have become more and more passively dependent on commercial suppliers. This is certainly also true of patrons of the food industry, who have tended more and more to be *mere* consumers—passive, uncritical, and dependent. Indeed, this sort of consumption may be said to be one of the chief goals of industrial production. The food industrialists have by now persuaded millions of consumers to prefer food that is already prepared. They will grow, deliver, and cook your food for you and (just like your mother) beg you to eat it. That they do not yet offer to insert it, prechewed, into your mouth is only because they have found no profitable way to do so. We may rest assured that they would be glad to find such a way. The ideal industrial food consumer would be strapped to a table with a tube running from the food factory directly into his or her stomach. (Think of the savings, the efficiency, and the effortlessness of such an arrangement!)

Perhaps I exaggerate, but not by much. The industrial eater is, in fact, one who does not know that eating is an agricultural act, who no longer knows or imagines the connections between eating and the land, and who is therefore necessarily passive and uncritical—in short, a victim. When food, in the minds of eaters, is no longer associated with farming and with the land, then the eaters are suffering a kind of cultural amnesia that is misleading and dangerous. The current version of the "dream home" of the future involves "effortless" shopping from a list of available goods on a television monitor and heating precooked food by remote control. Of course, this implies, and indeed depends on, a perfect ignorance of the history of the food that is consumed. It requires that the citizenry should give up their hereditary and sensible aversion to buying a pig in a poke. It wishes to make the selling of pigs in pokes an honorable and glamorous activity. The dreamer in this dream home will perforce know nothing about the kind or quality of this food, or where it came from, or how it was produced and prepared, or what ingredients, additives, and residues it contains. Unless, that is, the dreamer undertakes a close and constant study of the food industry, in which case he or she might as well wake up and play an active and responsible part in the economy of food.

There is, then, a politics of food that, like any politics, involves our freedom. We still (sometimes) remember that we cannot be free if our minds and voices are controlled by someone else. But we have neglected to understand that neither can we be free if our food and its sources are controlled by someone else. The condition of the passive consumer of food is not a democratic condition. One reason to eat responsibly is to live free.

But, if there is a food politics, there are also a food aesthetics and a food ethics, neither of which is dissociated from politics. Like industrial sex, industrial eating has become a degraded, poor, and paltry thing. Our kitchens and other eating places more and more resemble filling stations, as our homes more and more resemble motels. "Life is not very interesting," we seem to have decided. "Let its satisfactions be minimal, perfunctory, and fast." We hurry through our meals to go to work and hurry through our work in order to "recreate" ourselves in the evenings and on weekends and vacations. And then we hurry, with the greatest possible speed and noise and violence, through our recreation—for what? To eat the billionth hamburger at some fast-food joint hell-bent on increasing the "quality" of our life. And all this is carried out in a remarkable obliviousness of the causes and effects, the possibilities and the purposes of the life of the body in this world.

One will find this obliviousness represented in virgin purity in the advertisements of the food industry, in which the food wears as much makeup as the actors. If one gained one's whole knowledge of food—as some presumably do—from these advertisements, one would not know that the various edibles were ever living creatures, or that they all come from the soil, or that they were produced by work. The passive American consumer, sitting down to a meal of pre-prepared or fast food, confronts a platter covered with inert, anonymous substances that have been processed, dyed, breaded, sauced, gravied, ground, pulped, strained, blended, prettified, and sanitized beyond resemblance to any part of any creature that ever lived. The products of nature and agriculture have been made, to all appearances, the products of industry. Both eater and eaten are thus in exile from biological reality. And the result is a kind of solitude, unprecedented in human experience, in which the eater may think of eating as, first, a purely commercial transaction between him and a supplier, and then as a purely appetitive transaction between him and his food.

And this peculiar specialization of the act of eating is, again, of obvious benefit to the food industry, which has good reason to obscure the connection between food and farming. It would not do for the consumer to know that the hamburger she is eating came from a steer that spent much of its life standing deep in its own excrement in a feedlot, helping to pollute the local streams, or that the calf that yielded the veal cutlet on her plate spent its life in a box in which it did not have room to turn around. And, though her sympathy for the coleslaw might be less tender, she should not be encouraged to meditate on the hygienic and biological implications of mile-square fields of cabbage, for vegetables grown in huge monocultures are dependent on toxic chemicals just as animals in close confinement are dependent on antibiotics and other drugs.

The consumer, that is to say, must be kept from discovering that, in the food industry—as in any other industry—the over-riding concerns are not quality and health but volume and price. For decades now the entire industrial food economy, from the large farms and feedlots to the chains of fast-food restaurants and supermarkets, has been obsessed with volume. It has relentlessly increased scale in order to increase volume in order (presumably) to reduce costs. But, as scale increases, diversity declines; as diversity declines, so does health; as health declines, the dependence on drugs and chemicals necessarily increases. As capital replaces labor, it does so by substituting machines, drugs, and chemicals for human workers and for the natural health and fertility of the soil. The food is produced by any means or any shortcuts that will increase profits. And the business of the cosmeticians of advertising is to persuade the consumer that food so produced is good, tasty, healthful, and a guarantee of marital fidelity and long life.

It is, then, indeed possible to be liberated from the husbandry and wifery of the old household food economy. But one can be thus liberated only by entering a trap—unless one sees ignorance and helplessness, as many people apparently do, as the signs of privilege. The trap is the ideal of industrialism: a walled city surrounded by valves that let merchandise in but no consciousness out. How does one escape this trap? Only voluntarily, the same way that one went in—by restoring one's consciousness of what is involved in eating, by reclaiming responsibility for one's own part in the food economy. One might begin with Sir Albert Howard's illuminating principle that we should understand "the whole problem of health in soil, plant, animal, and man as one great subject." Eaters, that is, must understand that eating takes place inescapably in the world, that it is inescapably an agricultural act, and that how we eat determines, to a considerable extent, the way the world is used. This is a simple way of describing a relationship that is inexpressibly complex. To eat responsibly is to understand and enact, so far as one can, this complex relationship.

What can one do? Here is a list, probably not definitive:

Participate in food production to the extent that you can. If you have a yard or even just a porch box or a pot in a sunny window, grow something to eat in it. Make a little compost of your kitchen scraps, and use it for fertilizer. Only by growing some food for yourself can you become acquainted with the beautiful energy cycle that revolves from soil to seed to flower to fruit to food to offal to decay, and around again. You will be fully responsible for any food that you grow for yourself, and you will know all about it. You will appreciate it fully, having known it all its life.

Prepare your own food. This means reviving in your own mind and life the arts of kitchen and household. This should enable you to eat more cheaply and give you a measure of "quality control." You will have some reliable knowledge of what has been added to the food you eat.

Learn the origins of the food you buy, and buy the food that is produced closest to your home. The idea that every locality should be, as much as possible, the source of its own food makes several kinds of sense. The locally produced food supply is the most secure, the freshest, and the easiest for local consumers to know about and to influence.

Whenever you can, deal directly with a local farmer, gardener, or orchardist. All the reasons listed for the previous suggestion apply here. In addition, by such dealing, you eliminate the whole pack of merchants, transporters, processors, packagers, and advertisers who thrive at the expense of both producers and consumers.

Learn, in self-defense, as much as you can of the economy and technology of industrial food production. What is added to food that is not food, and what do you pay for these additions?

Learn what is involved in the *best* farming and gardening.

Learn as much as you can, by direct observation and experience if possible, of the life histories of the food species.

The last suggestion seems particularly important to me. Many people are now as much estranged from the lives of domestic plants and animals (except for flowers and dogs and cats) as they are from the lives of the wild ones. This is regrettable, for these domestic creatures are in diverse ways attractive; there is much pleasure in knowing them. And, at their best, farming, animal husbandry, horticulture, and gardening are complex and comely arts; there is much pleasure in knowing them, too.

And it follows that there is great displeasure in knowing about a food economy that degrades and abuses those arts and those plants and animals and the soil from which they come. For anyone who does know something of the modern history of food, eating away from home can be a chore. My own inclination is to eat seafood instead of red meat or poultry when I am traveling. Though I am by no means a vegetarian, I dislike the thought that some animal has been made miserable in order to feed me. If I am going to eat meat, I want it to be from an animal that has lived a pleasant, uncrowded life outdoors, on bountiful pasture, with good water nearby and trees for shade. And I am getting almost as fussy about food plants. I like to eat vegetables and fruits that I know have lived happily and healthily in good soil—not the products of the huge, bechemicaled factory-fields that I have seen, for example, in the Central Valley of California. The industrial farm is said to have been patterned on the factory production line. In practice, it invariably looks more like a concentration camp.

The pleasure of eating should be an *extensive* pleasure, not that of the mere gourmet. People who know the garden in which their vegetables have grown and know that the garden is healthy will remember the beauty of the growing plants, perhaps in the dewy first light of morning when gardens are at their best. Such a memory involves itself with the food and is one of the pleasures of eating. The knowledge of the good health of the garden relieves and frees and comforts the eater. The same goes for eating meat. The thought of the good pasture, and of the calf contentedly grazing, flavors the steak. Some, I know, will think it bloodthirsty or worse to eat a fellow creature you have known all its life. On the contrary, I think, it means that you eat with understanding and with gratitude. A significant part of the pleasure of eating is in one's accurate consciousness of the lives and the world from which food comes. The pleasure of eating, then, may be the best available standard of our health. And this pleasure, I think, is pretty fully available to the urban consumer who will make the necessary effort.

I mentioned earlier the politics, aesthetics, and ethics of food. But to speak of the pleasure of eating is to go beyond those categories. Eating with the fullest pleasure—pleasure, that is, that does not depend on ignorance—is perhaps the profoundest enactment of our connection with the world. In this pleasure we experience and celebrate our dependence and our gratitude, for we are living from mystery, from creatures we did not make and powers we cannot comprehend. When I think of the meaning of food, I always remember these lines by the poet William Carlos Williams, which seem to me merely honest:

There is nothing to eat,
　　　　seek it where you will,
　　　　　　　but the body of the Lord.
The blessed plants
　　　　and the sea, yield it
　　　　　　　to the imagination
　intact.

Making Sustainable Agriculture Work

Wes Jackson

In late June of this year, I watched boiling torrents of soil and water shoot through a six-foot-diameter culvert like water out of a nozzle to spray into a small creek in southeastern Nebraska. Rills quickly developed on the exposed fields and turned into gullies in a mere half-hour during what turned out to be a three-inch rain overnight. Stopping completely or inching along in my pickup, I watched all this and thought of well-fed and highly paid experts in our state colleges of agriculture, who still proclaim American agriculture a success story.

I wondered how there can be any talk of success in farming when such huge amounts of ecological capital erode seaward. For that matter, what kind of education is it where researchers routinely apply the discoveries of Charles Darwin and Gregor Mendel in order to increase yield and build insect and pathogen resistance but ignore the implications of placing chemicals into the environment—chemicals with which our tissues and those of our livestock have no evolutionary experience, chemicals that should be regarded as guilty until proven innocent? Is nature to be subdued or ignored in the interest of agricultural production? Should the goal of farming and agricultural research be to increase the productive capacity of our various crops and livestock? Should agriculture serve as an instrument for the expansion of industry? We might find ourselves appalled at a positive answer to any of these questions, but, turned into statements, they are in fact the assumptions of modern agriculture.

Subdue or ignore nature; increase production; use agriculture as an instrument for the expansion of industry—what are the consequences of these assumptions? Nature is dominated or ignored with each plowing and chemical application. By emphasizing increased production, we have narrowed the germ plasm of our crops and livestock. Use of a bovine growth hormone, for example, promises a 30 percent increase in milk production; meanwhile, a Cornell University study predicts up to a 30 percent reduction in the number of dairy farmers. Cows will have fewer lactations before slaughter, for calcium is apparently sucked from the bones of hormone-treated cows faster than the rate of biological replacement. Thus, calcium deficiency diseases are now anticipated. The only good to come from such consequences is that the job of the animal rights activists may become easier.

Scientists with the U.S. Department of Agriculture recently spliced a human growth hormone gene into swine. These hogs gain faster and are leaner, satisfying both the commercial grower and the yuppie, but they are arthritic and cross-eyed. Such problems are regarded primarily as simple aspects of fine-tuning the hog. Meanwhile, hogs receiving the bovine growth hormone may be leaner and gain faster, but they experience gastric ulcers, renal disease, dermatitis, and an enlarged heart, as well as arthritis. The justification for these experiments again arises from the assumption that the goal of farming and agricultural research should be to increase the productive capacity of our various crops and livestock. The monsters created by such applications of biotechnology are perhaps the humans who see nothing wrong with making animals miserable.

As recent as it is, the third assumption—that agriculture is to serve as an instrument for the expansion of industry—is already deeply ingrained in the American mind. The secretary of agriculture, who has become little more than the administrative assistant or deputy to the secretary of commerce, participates in a national policy of food for export, not so much to help farmers but as a way to offset the balance-of-payments deficit in order to buy, among other things, foreign oil. In the late 1970s, we exported as much as $45 billion worth of food.

But the most dramatic statement I have seen that reflects the assumption that agriculture is to remain an instrument for industrial expansion was made in 1982 by Orville Bentley, former dean of the College of Agriculture at the University of Illinois and then assistant secretary for science and education in the

USDA. Bentley announced a rapid change to mobilize our resources toward biotechnology, including genetic manipulation. He argued that this would happen as "a way to keep the level of technology high." This motivation, to keep the level of technology high, is orders of magnitude worse than "art for art's sake," for it operates at the expense of farm families and rural communities. Bentley's statement betrays our nation's adherence to the third assumption. Farmers themselves are not considered.

The biotechnology craze will die down someday, partly because, like earlier crazes in biology, the payoffs will disappoint the proponents and investors. Furthermore, I think we will see a growing uncertainty about the ecological consequences of altered organisms. Proper assessment will require understanding biology at all levels—a prospect that any biologist who has taught general biology will find discouraging. Biotechnology is an issue, dropped into our laps, that already requires countless hours of thinking, reading, and discussion. The conscientious citizen now has even less time to enjoy the world. We can hope that it will soon become apparent that the rewards of biotechnology will run mostly to the suppliers of inputs—the Monsantos and others—not to the farmer and the landscape.

Taken together, these three assumptions directly threaten Thomas Jefferson's vision of a nation of farmers and free citizens as the best bet for a healthy democracy. Those of us who suggest that we abandon or greatly modify these three assumptions are often accused of nostalgia. But what if Chautauqua-type meetings were held around the country where small groups of five, twenty-five, fifty, or a hundred and more would address the basic question: Is the Jeffersonian ideal of the family farm and strong rural community mere nostalgia or a practical necessity in a world of declining energy and material resources?

If our bottom-line goal is an assured food supply into a distant future, how are we to protect what is needed to achieve it? Soil erosion will have to be reduced to natural replacement levels. Dependency on petroleum will have to end, and the water supplies for humans and livestock will have to receive a drastically reduced rate of alien chemicals. Biological nitrogen fixation will have to replace nitrogen fertilizer made from natural

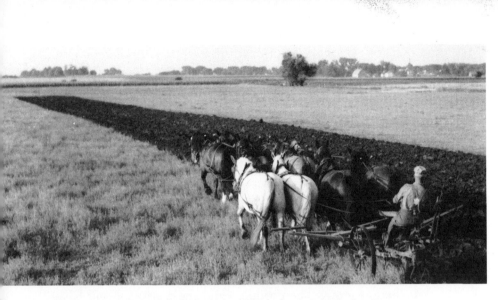

Plowing, Hardin County, Iowa, September 1939. Photo by Arnold Rothstein.

gas, which means that crop rotations involving legumes will have to return. Since the crumb structure found in healthy soils is enhanced by animal manure, we will have to get animals back on the farm and out of commercial feedlots in order to help our soils and save energy. To conserve our agricultural base for the long run, in other words, we must insist that our farms meet certain ecological standards similar to those we see in natural ecosystems, such as prairies. The key is to feature diversity *and* a manageable scale—a high eyes-to-acres ratio. Not everyone, of course, but millions of people must return to the land if we are ever to place agriculture back on its biological feet.

Our bottom-line goal of increased production has been too narrow, and, when a bottom line is so narrow, it can only accommodate short-run profit. That's the bottom line that will break the system.

In addition to considering people and land, we must also think about community. Rural communities must be large enough that the family farm is as much a derivative of the community as a contributor to it. Without community, the subsidies and profits that farm families receive go on immediately to the suppliers of inputs and to the cities. We need small businesses to intercept that money where it can roll over and over long enough to support rural schools, rural churches, rural baseball.

The corporate farm simply uses the extractive economy of agribusiness as a profit-only enterprise with little interest in the potentially renewable economy of agriculture. But, on a corporate farm, who watches the land under cultivation, especially land that slopes? Who takes seriously the slow knowledge, the accumulated mistakes and successes over generations? If land is to serve as more than an instrument for yielding a simple cipher in a quarterly report, it will need sympathy and love. In short, a seamless web of people, land, and community is all that will satisfy the ecological and cultural requirements for a sustainable agriculture.

But there is more: The producer and the consumer will have to confront one another in a dialectical manner. The necessary transition cannot begin until we as a people, both in the cities and the country, embrace the Jeffersonian idea that the nation's strength indeed depends on the "free man" on the land. This is not some archaic, two-hundred-year-old idea whose utility has vanished. It was an old idea two hundred years ago, an idea central to western civilization almost from the beginning. It was there with the Hebrews at Mount Sinai, with the desert and Egypt behind them, as they looked forward to the Promised Land of Canaan where each person would sit under one's own fig tree, have one's own vineyard, and be one's own priest. This democratic ideal, thankfully, is also an ecological ideal, for it accommodated the possibility and necessity that many people paid close attention to what Thoreau called "meeting the expectations of the land."

I hope all of us understand that none of this necessarily means a return to provincialism. The land can't hold everyone, but those who do return to it can, if they desire, enjoy French wine, Russian novels, Greek philosophy, and Tuscan cooking. Those who do return to the land—who choose to raise their children somewhere other than in shopping malls—in my view increase the chances for respecting other people, a respect that goes beyond toleration. Our turning to our own places, if the scale of those places is right, should enhance our wish that others may experience similar blessings of justice and liberty. But what will this take?

I think a big idea is beginning to emerge in the American mind. It is becoming apparent that our problem with the earth is the result of our "subdue-and-ignore" assumptions, assumptions not just about agriculture but about everything else. We have assumed control of nature without adequately understanding nature's arrangements. In the case of agriculture, we have tried to understand it by looking almost exclusively to what industry has had to offer. But a few are saying that, since nature has the most sustainable ecosystems and since ultimately agriculture comes out of nature, our standard for a sustainable world should be nature's own ecosystems. "Nature as the measure," "nature as an analogy," "nature as the standard"—these are some of the phrases to think about in hopes that an expanding number of agriculturists and ecologists will begin to explore seriously the possibility of a marriage between ecology and agriculture, including agricultural science.

It won't be the first time, of course, that humans have advocated that we return to nature as our primary teacher. Wendell Berry has traced some of the literary history of this idea from Job into the early part of the nineteenth century.[1] The notion disappears from English literature apparently after Alexander Pope. When it surfaces again, it is among scientists— Liberty Hyde Bailey, J. Russell Smith, and Sir Albert Howard, among others.

Our work at the Land Institute in Salina, Kansas, began in 1976. In 1978 I published a paper in which I suggested that the native prairie be our standard, based on the assumption that the best agriculture mimics natural ecosystems. Since then, our small group of researchers has set out to build domestic prairies that would produce perennial grains grown in mixtures as substitutes for annual monocultures on hillsides. Our time frame is the range from twenty-five to a hundred years. Our work, however, had its origin *ignorant* of a literary and scientific tradition; as Wendell Berry said about those poets and scientists, their understanding probably came out of the "familial and communal handing down in the agrarian common culture, rather than in any succession of teachers and students in the literary culture or in the schools." I know that I, for one, was ignorant of the literary and scientific history. Instead, the ideas expressed in that 1978 paper were probably inspired by my background in biology, a love for prairie, and my farm upbringing, giving me a "memory" embedded in that agrarian common culture. I don't know, really. Walt Whitman has said that "perfect memory is perfect forgetfulness." To know something well is to not know where it came from.

The big idea of "nature as the measure" acknowledges the respect necessary to modify greatly (if not abandon) the current assumptions surrounding modern agriculture. In the 1978 paper that established the paradigm for our research, the assumption was that we must begin with the prairie because that was what was here. I also asked, "What will nature require?" Since then we have added a third consideration, embedded in the first two: "What will nature help us to do here?" Berry has pointed out that, as we cut the forests and plowed the great prairies, "We have never known what we were doing because we have never known what we were undoing." A future agriculture will require that we learn as much as possible about what we undid.

Astronaut Edgar Mitchell has often been asked what it was like to experience the moon. He replies that he was "too busy being operational to experience the moon." Life on the moon requires the ultimate in instrumentation to keep the little earth-environment of the astronaut functioning.

As we employ our knowledge to accommodate our demands and to tinker with the earth, we create acid rain, deplete the ozone, contaminate groundwater, and perhaps cause global warming. Increasingly, we are taking conscious measures to protect ourselves from the problems we create; thus, we have become increasingly busy and "more operational," with less and less time to *experience* the earth. Many people want to be astronauts; the way the earth is deteriorating, perhaps the astronauts will be the sole survivors. If only Mission Earth could become our space program . . .

Such sober thoughts can create sober people. But we have to

be careful, for we can become so frightened that we make it our full-time job to save the earth. Some have done just that, denying themselves the time to enjoy the very earth they are trying to save. Doing so, they lose the sight and feeling for what they are supposedly saving. Edward Abbey said it best a short time before his death last March: "Be a half-assed crusader, a part-time fanatic. Don't worry too much about the fate of the world. Saving the world is only a hobby. Get out there and enjoy the world, your girlfriend, your boyfriend, husbands, wives; climb mountains, run rivers, get drunk, do whatever you want to do while you can, before it's too late."

"Toward a Sustainable Agriculture" is the title I chose for my 1978 article; I don't remember why precisely, but I do remember thinking about the word "permanent" and rejecting it as not correct for an ever-changing earth. I am sure I am not the first person to use the term *sustainable agriculture* in print, although some have credited me with doing so. The concept and the term have now become widespread in the common culture. But what does sustainable agriculture mean today?

William Lockeretz has recently summarized much of the discussion on the subject, citing the various concepts that now surround the term and the ways in which it has evolved.[2] Lockeretz makes a bold attempt to deal with what he calls some of the "fundamental questions." After considering the differences among sustainable, alternative, low-input, ecological, and regenerative agriculture, he goes on to raise and then address the following questions:

Is sustainable agriculture in the United States primarily a matter of reducing certain inputs, or reducing inputs in general, or instituting positive practices that make some inputs unnecessary?

Does sustainable agriculture require fundamental changes either in the economic and institutional environment or in farmers' motivations and values?

Does understanding sustainable agriculture involve concepts that are fundamentally different from conventional systems, or do we only need to extend the application of known principles to the conditions that prevail under sustainable practices?

To what extent do the resource-conserving and environmentally sounder techniques being developed at mainstream agricultural institutions already represent sustainable agriculture?

Does sustainable agriculture require a higher level of management ability among farmers?

These are important questions, but a definition that might arise out of a constellation of answers to such questions is likely to miss the point. As the sustainable-agriculture effort unfolds, it is becoming increasingly clear that "sustainable" is a complex political word. Political terms are especially vulnerable to co-optation, to the point that the term could be used as a weapon by proponents of large-scale industrialized agribusiness, people who want agriculture to go on as it is now. Like most political words, "sustainable" is vulnerable to the effects of both history and passion, making it even more important that we remember its origins and recall that the term does not come out of the re-search plots of the government experimental stations or the private agribusiness companies. We cannot, therefore, allow it to be defined by such people or, for that matter, only by farmers. More accurately, the word comes from the few people in the common culture who are frustrated with the extractive economy and the desecration of the land and water that sustain agriculture. Our understanding of the word may change, but it will retain a core of meanings, a core that will have importance proportional to the amount of care and practice it deserves. And herein lies the challenge, for only care and practice can keep it healthy. In that sense, it is like other words that express our ideals—words such as justice, truth, beauty, love.

An irate member of an audience at a land-grant university once asked me for my definition of sustainable agriculture and stated that "it had better be in ten words or less or I am not going to listen." I could not accommodate him. Reaching into the core of my understanding, I found myself using such words as diversity, conservation, balance, scale.

So, since it is a political term, political education will be as important as education in proper field techniques. The proper teachers will be those who start with the assumption that we are mostly *ignorant* of how to do sustainable agriculture, an assumption that will stand over and against the assumptions of modern agriculture, which is based on knowledge, not ignorance. Descartes's discourse on methods carries this statement: "It seemed to me that the effort to instruct myself had no effect other than the increasing discovery of my own ignorance." Rather than regard this, as Wendell Berry put it, as "an apt description of the human condition, and a very proper result of an education,"[3] the culture at large, including conventional agriculturists, tends to agree with Descartes that this situation is correctable. The other side, those who look to nature for a standard, more likely agrees with Berry that it is not correctable, believing instead that, since we are basically ignorant about eventual outcomes, it is best to be students of the way the world has worked.

Teachers of sustainable agriculture, be they organic farmers, environmental activists, or university professors and researchers, may feel inclined toward both self-righteousness ("We are farming without chemicals" and "We are farming nature's way") and self-pity ("We do all this extra work so that we won't have to use the chemicals, yet we are not properly compensated for our labor"). Both attitudes will have to be avoided at all costs. We are all in this together, and, if we are to be like the best of political educators, our words must reflect the *reality* of our common predicament. This may not be easy, especially when our strongest urges are to remain distant and feel superior. But, when it comes to sustaining life on earth, loving our enemies is not some hollow morality; it is a practical necessity.

Notes

1. Wendell Berry, "Poetry and Place" in *Standing by Words: Essays by Wendell Berry* (San Francisco: North Point Press, 1983), p. 106.

2. William Lockeretz, "Open Questions in Sustainable Agriculture," *Journal of Alternative Agriculture* 3, no. 4 (1989), pp. 174–81.

3. Personal communication to the author.

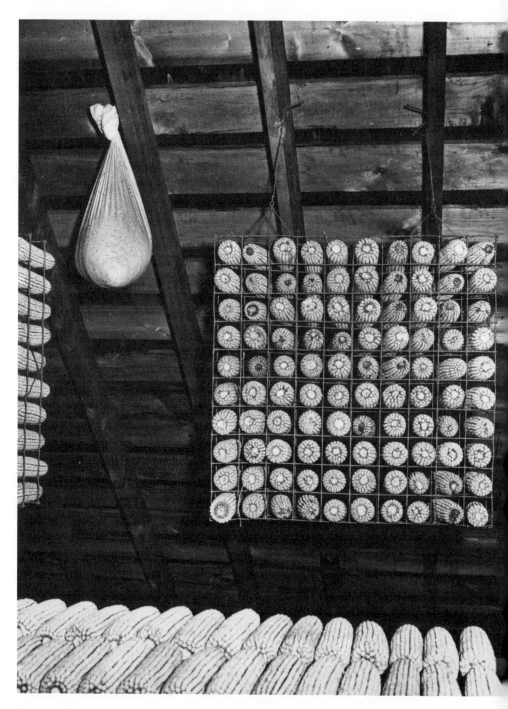

Open-pollinated Seed Corn, Marshall City, Iowa, October 1939. Photo by
Arnold Rothstein.

Food, Farming, and Democracy
Frances Moore Lappé

A bumper sticker appeared midway through the farm crisis of
the 1980s that said, "If you eat, you're involved in agriculture."
It seems an uncontroversial proposition: Food comes from
farms; all of us need food; therefore, we all have an interest in
farming. It's nevertheless a connection that most of us have
difficulty making. Farmers look increasingly like yet one more
special-interest group. Despite what we may rationally know, our
daily experience tells us that food comes from a supermarket.
We are removed, physically and psychically, from the farm. At
the same time, as consumers we seem to be growing more and
more dissatisfied with our food: We worry about its purity,
wholesomeness, and healthfulness; we are disappointed with its
flavor and quality; and we sense that mealtimes — the experience
of preparing and sharing food — seem to lack the feeling of
hearth and home, of family and community, that they once had,
or that we imagine they once had.

So perhaps it's not surprising that, as a society, we seem unable to resolve either our farm crisis — a crisis that has arguably
been continuous since the 1930s — or our dissatisfaction with our
food. We don't really see the connection between the two, and so
are unable to develop what must be an integrated solution to
what is really one problem. Our imaginations and ability to
create solutions are therefore impaired: We cannot move toward
a future we cannot imagine, and we cannot imagine a future we
don't believe is possible. The aim of this essay is to ask each of
us to search our hearts and our minds in order to discover a
vision of food and farming we *can* believe in — one we can
believe in because it faces and embraces the practical and logical

consequences of what both our deepest intuitions and our most unrelenting analyses tell us. But wishful thinking is the opposite of what I mean by "imagining a future." Rather, we must in our mind's eye be able to see a system of food production and consumption here in the United States that could genuinely work for the people and for the land—not just on a few oddball farms but on all farms—a system that is environmentally, economically, and culturally sustainable as well as genuinely democratic. Such a vision must begin with the principle of a sustainable agriculture, an agriculture consistent with the long-term well-being of both people and the land.

Powerful cultural messages, however, form and deform our view of what is possible. Take the "family farm," a term that already has a quaint ring to it and is surely taken seriously only by those who are out of step. Those who believe in the family farm may be right in some moral sense, but progress does not stop for the sentimental. When, four years ago, liberal farm analysts Susan Sechler and Ken Cook wrote an influential article under the title "It's Time to Face the Facts: The Family Farm Is Doomed," they were just stating the obvious in the eyes of most Americans.[1] Still, most of us continue to give lip service to the notion of the family farm, to the Jeffersonian ideal of an agrarian America. But few of us have a glimmering of the real social, economic, and political context in which such an agriculture and such a society could flourish. We are prevented from imagining a workable framework for these things because, in my view, they would—by definition—require a democratic economy. The historian Lawrence Goodwyn wrote: "We have two languages, one rooted in Adam Smith and one rooted in Karl Marx. Neither provides a theory of the democratic state. . . . You can't create a society you can't imagine. And if you can't imagine a democratic society, you can't have one."[2]

I believe Goodwyn is right. We have no language with which to conceive of a democratic society or agriculture. But our biggest stumbling block may be that we have been made to believe that we don't need to conceive of one. "Free-market" agriculture is *by definition* a democratic agriculture, isn't it? They are one and the same. With this view, we needn't bother ourselves with imagining and then creating a democratic economy. By "free-market" agriculture I mean an economy driven by an exchange of commodities, including farmland and labor, based on market prices. I mean an economy not just based on private property but one allowing unlimited individual accumulation of even the scarcest resources. I mean an economy in which labor and ownership are almost universally distinct. While we associate these rules with a democratic economy, they are, especially in agriculture, inadequate tools.

Left to its own devices, the market leads to concentration of control. In agriculture, this reality has special significance. Because industry and trade (compared to farming) lend themselves more readily to concentration, farmers today find they are squeezed between two highly organized sectors—what economists call "oligopolistic" industries. On one side are the manufacturers of farm supplies and equipment, from pesticides to combines, along with the banking industry. On the other are the trade and processing industries. In each, a handful of companies command the field.

Such oligopolies can pass on their increased costs to customers, including farmers, thus assuring themselves a profit. But farmers have to swallow increased costs—especially those farmers not big enough to skirt the market through bulk discount buying and other devices. And they have to take whatever price traders and processors offer. Farmers who want to remain competitive cannot pass on their increased costs by hiking their prices.

Thus, where the market governs, it's not surprising that an imbalance in power (and therefore in reward) develops between primary food producers and industrial behemoths. But the problem with the market is not just that such gross inequities allow some to protect their profits at the expense of others. The problem is the price mechanism itself. Price is the only information the market offers, and it is grossly deficient. Commodity prices, to which all producers in a market must respond to stay in business, do not incorporate the true *resource* or *human* costs of production. Nor do prices include the cost of (and therefore alert us to) the erosion of topsoil or the drawing down of groundwater reserves. Neither do they reflect the difficulties passed to later generations who must grow food on impoverished soil with depleted groundwater. In the "free" market, what nature makes has no price. It is "free."

Closely related prices of farm inputs—fertilizers, pesticides, machinery—also send farmers false signals. The market says: Any machine that increases income this year is a good deal. The market cannot warn farmers that the choice may be generating a dependency that will threaten their economic survival when their neighbors buy the same machine, pushing production up and commodity prices down. Neither can the market inform farmers that their choice of certain inputs may heighten their risk of contracting our most deadly forms of cancer.

There is yet another problem with price as the measure of the health of farming. Prices of commodities tell us nothing about whose pockets ultimately get lined from the farmers' labor. Commodity prices multiplied by volume make up gross farm sales, not what farmers actually get to keep. Since 1940, adjusted for inflation, the *gross* income of the farming sector taken as a whole has doubled, largely because of vast increases in volume.[3] At the same time, net income from farming has fallen by 10 percent. In other words, more than the equivalent of the entire increase in income to farmers since 1940 has gone *not to farmers* themselves but to manufacturers of farm supplies and to banks. Commodity prices and farm output really tell us little about what the farming sector ultimately ends up with. And, within the farm sector, three-fourths of net farm income ends up in the hands of a mere 5 percent of farmers.

My point is simple: The market price simply cannot provide the information needed to protect both the land and the people who farm it. It ignores vital information—the costs to land, soil, and human health—on which our ultimate survival depends. It is blind to other critical questions: whether gross returns from farm sales actually remain on the farm and, a parallel question within the farm sector, which farmers (a few or the vast majority?) enjoy the gains from greater volume or better prices.

The market and its prices might play a constructive role were it not for the second rule of the market economy that undermines sustainable agriculture: Capitalism divides owner-ship from work. In 1986, almost 40 percent of farmland sales went to city investors such as doctors and lawyers, doubling their typical share of the farmland market.[4] As a speculative commodity, wealth—not land wisdom—becomes the criterion for ownership. Farmland ownership is thus severed from the culture of agriculture, from the body of knowledge and skills that grows out of generations on the land.

In a market economy, labor is strictly a commodity as well. Farmland has increasingly become the domain of the wealthy; by the 1980s, for the first time in American history, most of the work on farms was being done by hired labor. Agriculture dependent on hired labor belies the vision of sustainable agriculture. Sustainable agriculture is necessarily knowledge-intensive, depending on *all* the faculties of the farmer. Since sustainable agriculture consists of a mix of crops together with livestock, farmers must understand the many interrelations of their chosen mix to enrich the soil and minimize pest damage.

In short, sustainable agriculture depends on a specific type of relationship of the farmer to the land. It must be an enduring one, for only over time can the necessary knowledge be acquired. And the farmer must feel a personal stake in the welfare of the land to call forth not just the physical exertion required but also the mental alertness needed to observe and record subtle changes and interactions over decades. Such a relationship is incompatible with farm labor as a commodity and with farm ownership as an investment. Price—the compelling determinant in market relationships—is a wholly insufficient and often misleading guide to land use or indicator of a fair return to most farmers. And land and labor treated as mere commodities necessarily dissociate agriculture from the culture that sustains it. By contrast, a democratic agriculture would depend in large measure on a set of noneconomic relationships, on rules and values in direct conflict with those economic relationships just described.

In a sustainable agriculture, which rules and values would hold? For one, land is not an investment, returning income by virtue of inflation to an owner who does nothing. Land is a *tool* with which to earn a living by working it well. Land, however, is not a tool *exclusively:* It has value in and of itself. Because of its intrinsic worth and its value to unborn generations, a farmer seeks not to maximize output from the land but to leave the land "more valuable at the end of his life than it was when he took hold of it," in Theodore Roosevelt's words.[5] And, in a sustainable agriculture, land is not just a place to live, interchangeable within any urban site. It is a locus of enriched family life because, almost uniquely in today's world, it offers the possibility of shared economic responsibilities within the family.

Thus, over the life of our nation, to the degree that our farmers have embodied (or imagined themselves to embody) any of these values, they have never fit the market model. To some degree, the culture of agriculture has always been a culture apart from its economic structure. Little by little, however, the fit has gotten better and better. Farmers and nonfarmers alike have watched as capitalist economic rules have steadily eroded the very essence of family-farm agriculture—dispersed, diversified, family-owned-and-operated farming. We have watched the values underpinning that culture increasingly violated: our sense of the sacred desecrated as topsoil is lost and groundwater contaminated; our sense of justice trammeled as the most economically powerful, rather than the most conscientious or hardworking, reap the biggest rewards; our sense of caring for each other— love itself—devalued as we are asked to accept our neighbor's demise. It's just the market's discipline at work weeding out the inefficient, we're told. It might hurt, but, in the end, it's good for us all. With this understanding, it's easier to see why farming in America, along with its satisfactions, has been a plain of conflict, disappointment, and pain for so many.

Much of this we all know. But, as shoppers, cooks, and partakers of food, we labor under the same assumptions about the market economy and its benefits as we do about agriculture— assumptions that blind us not only to the real problems of food producers but also to our own plight as food consumers. As in agriculture, price dominates all discussion of food consumption. Since 1945 and the beginnings of "agribusiness," the American experience of food and eating has been largely quantitative rather than qualitative. We point with pride to how little of our income we spend on food, how much we produce, and how little time we spend preparing or eating it. If flavor, purity, and the psychological and social satisfactions of food disappear in the process, that must be weighed against the clear economic miracle that is the system of contemporary American food production and consumption. It is, we are told, surely a small price to pay. As of 1987, according to the U.S. Department of Agriculture, Americans spent less than 10 percent of their disposable income on food—a record. I want to suggest that in fact the price we pay is very high indeed—that in fact we pay dearly as individuals and as a society for the way in which we presently produce and consume food.

We have already seen how our food production system harms all but the largest farms and how it damages our environment, our land, and our rural communities. Cheap food has been made possible at the farmer's expense, not at the expense of the food processor or distributor, who receives 75 percent of every dollar spent on food.[6] The economic miracle of today's cheap American food has involved a colossal transfer of income and capital from producers to middlemen—to the agricultural equivalents of Wall Street arbitrageurs and bond sellers. In the third world, large plantations of cash crops grown for export by multinationals or local elites tend to reinforce both the concentration of land and wealth in a few hands and the continuing powerlessness of ordinary people. Displacing the variety of crops necessary to sustain the local population, monocultures of fruit and vegetables grown for the out-of-season market in America ensure that we will not go without cheap and varied food year-round. But they also increase the wealth of elite landholders, providing the wherewithal for their further expansion. And our appetite for meat—meat that we don't need and that may in fact be harming our health—contributes not only to the overproduction of feed grain at the expense of other crops but also to the conversion of rain forest to grazing land and thus to global warming.

Even if we choose to ignore the effects of our food production system on others, we ourselves pay for it in ways that most of us can only begin to comprehend. In our supposedly cheap food are hidden costs that we pay for once as consumers and then again as taxpayers. Our tax dollars not only pay for agricultural subsidies (which, like virtually everything else in contemporary agribusiness, benefit the wealthiest the most) but also provide irrigation water and energy at unconscionable discounts to large growers. We also fund the USDA and the land-grant college system, agencies originally designed to support all farmers but that now dedicate their energies almost exclusively to aiding large agribusiness operations. And even those government entities explicitly set up to protect and help us as consumers seem reluctant to pursue any course that goes against the interest of big agriculture and food processing: In the recent outcry over Alar, for example, government has been the *last* to act, following well on the heels of the apple industry and Alar's manufacturer. In a price-fixated, market-driven food and farming system, the government seems unable or unwilling to deal with consumer concerns about food safety and purity.

There are other, perhaps less dramatic, costs. The flavor of our food has suffered as a result of varieties developed not for their inherent aesthetic qualities but for the convenience of growers, distributors, and processors. And, next to cost, we have been sold on convenience as the highest virtue. The value of the fast food most of us eat away from home or the convenience food we heat or microwave in our own kitchens lies almost entirely in its convenience, its uniformity, and its capacity to save us time — time presumably to be spent earning more money or buying more consumer goods. Since human beings are adaptable creatures, we become convinced that tomatoes in February really are worth eating, that heating processed food in a microwave oven is cooking, and that fast-food and chain restaurants are an adequate substitute for the pleasure, community, and solace that traditional restaurant and family meals once gave us. This aesthetic desensitization also assists in distancing us yet further from the realities of where and how our food is produced. And so, in the market economy, the process comes full circle. We are its perpetrators and simultaneously its victims.

Why, it must be asked, do we accept these trends—trends that even you who do not accept my analysis of their relation to the market economy might still find unsatisfactory from so many points of view? Could it be because of a belief system that we ourselves already hold? I believe the answer, unfortunately, is yes. It is a belief system that allows us to avoid admitting the many obvious ways in which the market violates our deepest values. As long as we cannot admit, or even see, how the market/commodity rules violate us, we will lack the motivation and courage to resist.

We avoid seeing or admitting the impact of market economy through a mental packaging of our ideas about ourselves. The essential trick is believing that we are each really two people— one "moral" and one "economic." And entirely different rules apply to these two different entities within. Let's take our "economic self" first. For two hundred years, Jeremy Bentham's utilitarianism and a distorted version of Adam Smith's economic philosophy have been used to teach us that by nature we are cold, calculating economic rationalists, weighing every choice in relation to how it furthers our narrow self-interest.

In the last decade, the emerging field of sociobiology— pioneered by E. O. Wilson's study of the biological determinants of human social behavior—has been misread to entrench this view of ourselves. The notion of a "selfish gene" (from Richard Dawkins's 1976 book by that title) has further reinforced the notion of individuals as calculating atoms, each out for its own good. And biotechnology, with its capacity to "invent" and now patent new life, has further diminished our view of ourselves. Such a self-image melds perfectly with the market metaphor of free-ranging economic entities wheeling and dealing in purely economic exchanges. So, while our religious leaders often warn that our problem is hubris, that we mortals have an overly exalted sense of ourselves, I fear an opposite problem. We have an increasingly *dismal* view of ourselves. As an "economic self," one is simply an instinct-driven, self-interested collection of genes. It's worth noting that such a view of life is relatively new. Marshall Sahlins, author of *The Use and Abuse of Biology,* has written: "So far as I am aware, we are the only society that thinks of itself as having risen from savagery, identified with a ruthless nature. Everyone else believes they are descended from gods."[7]

On the other hand, opposed to this economic self, many Americans still cling to a belief in a "moral self." Even if not churchgoers, most Americans report that they believe in God and in religious virtues. Therefore, if pressed, most of us would no doubt proclaim a belief in the possibility of unselfish love, fellow feeling, and cooperation. But my point is that such a view of ourselves, if it exists at all, exists in increasing subordination to that of the "economic self." Human beings seek internal consistency. It's exceedingly difficult to maintain the notion that we are "moral beings" on Sunday and when we put the kids to bed at night but are "economic beings" the rest of the week. Seeking unity, we let the "economic self" increasingly define our entirety.

I see evidence of this progression all around. While renting out one's body for another's sexual pleasure has always seemed aberrant—reducing intimacy to an economic exchange— relatively few people today are speaking out against a much greater affront to our internal unity: so-called surrogate motherhood. Is it not because the renting of wombs and the selling of infants become perfectly consistent once we have become an "economic self"? So now I have a tentative answer to my earlier question: Why do we tolerate rules of economic life that violate our sense of the sacred, of justice, of love itself? Because, perhaps, in our hearts we seriously doubt that these rules do in fact violate our nature at all. We've come to believe that the commodity/market system, rather than violating our nature, handily conforms to, or even reflects, our dominant nature.

That is the problem. Capitalist rules belie a sustainable agriculture and run roughshod over values long associated with family-farm agriculture—rules we tolerate despite the fact that they violate our deepest beliefs. Similarly, those same rules play havoc with the wholesomeness and pleasure we ought to expect from our food. We experience ourselves as two people—as a walking, talking dualism. Since our feeling, caring selves can't be heard above the dominant voice of our economic selves, we come to belittle the violation of our values. If an "economic being" is who we *really* are, we lack the conviction to withstand the intimidation of those who defend the market rules regardless of their impact. We lack courage. We acquiesce.

How can we resolve our imagined dualism driven by our "economic selves"? I'll make only a few suggestions. Our religious traditions surely offer guidance. Unfortunately, however, for many people institutional religion has reinforced the notion that economic life and moral life are separate realms. And the recent debacle of TV evangelists only illustrates the startling degree to which religion has been taken over by economic values. In contrast, the Catholic bishops' pastoral letter on the American economy, "Economic Justice for All," and comparable teachings now emerging from the Protestant churches reverse that trend. Theirs are courageous calls for a rejection of the "economic self" and a reunification of ourselves from the other direction, by infusing moral values into economic life.

We can buttress these initiatives. We can, in addition, reclaim a philosophic heritage long denied us. Today Adam Smith's authority is used to confirm our selfish nature. We hear only of Smith's *Wealth of Nations,* that famous 1776 treatise proposing that our self-interest operates as an "invisible hand" to the benefit of all. Forgotten is Smith's *Theory of Moral Sentiments* in which he argues that human behavior is grounded in an *innate* morality. The work begins: "How selfish soever man may be supposed, there are evidently some principles in his nature which interest him in the fortune of others, and render their happiness necessary to him, though he derives nothing from it except the pleasure of seeing it."[8] Adam Smith saw no dualism. We are *social* by our very nature. He wrote, "It is thus that man, who can subsist only in society, was fitted by nature to that situation for which he was made."[9] We cannot escape our concern for the well-being of others.

Just as Adam Smith's wisdom has been consistently reduced to reinforce the notion of the narrow "economic self," so Charles Darwin's work has been misused to teach false lessons about our competitive, selfish nature. Didn't Darwin believe we all evolved in a dog-eat-dog world where "survival of the fittest" was the unpleasant truth pushing evolution along? Overlooked has been

Darwin's insight that natural selection favored altruism, cooperation, and mutual aid. Darwin wrote: "As man advances in civilization and small tribes are united into larger communities, the simplest reason would tell each individual that he ought to extend his social instinct and sympathies to all members of the same nation, though personally unknown to him." [10]

Interpretations of modern sociobiology assume that this new theory just takes Darwin one step further, arguing that it is the *gene,* not the particular organism, that must perpetuate itself in order for evolution to make sense. What is missed is a profound irony: "Selfish" genes create "unselfish" entities. Because, for genes to survive, the organisms of which they are a part must serve the survival not just of themselves but also of all other entities with the same genes. Such theories can begin to explain the cooperation and self-sacrifice found throughout nature and through human evolution. They help us understand how such behaviors could predate formal social rules imposing cooperation from the outside or even predate what Darwin called the "simplest reason." Thus, even modern-day sociobiology—the bane of many humanists—actually suggests a biological, genetic basis for fellow feeling and altruism, one on which (it could be argued) culture can build ever broader circles of caring to include more and more of our cohabitants on this small planet. [11]

I have taken this excursion not, of course, to try to convince you that human beings by nature have a great capacity for caring and selflessness. Rather, I have tried to point out that we live in a culture deeply imbued with the opposite view of our nature, a dualistic view in which the economic self rules. My contention is this: Only as we leave behind this false notion of the "economic self" will we be able to critique and resist economic rules that violate our deepest intuitions about our most basic human values and needs, including the three I mentioned earlier: our need to cherish the sacred (including our land), our need for fairness as the very basis of community, and our need for love expressed in solidarity with our neighbors. More than acquisitors, we are creators, developers of our unique capacities. More than isolated egos, we are social beings in search of meaningful communities. This is our essence.

From such a vantage point, we can look afresh at received economic dogma. We are free to view the market and private property, not as the be-all and end-all, not as the definition of democratic economic life, but simply as what they are: devices that we can *use* to create economies serving healthy, satisfying communities. Understanding human beings as developers of innate gifts, we can place emphasis in a democratic agricultural economy not on maximum acquisition but on maximum opportunity. Such an agricultural economy seeks to enable as many people as possible to apply their talents to farming. A farm economy reflecting such a view of our nature and responding to the values I have outlined might set these parameters: First, farmers alone own farmland—not bankers, insurance companies, or landlords. This is possible only if farmers are able to pay for farmland solely with the income they earn from farming it. And this is possible only if farmers in each new generation must pay for the land by farming it. In such a vision, the market and private property do have roles to play: determining roles, not supportive ones. They are seen not as values in themselves but as devices in the service of moral values.

Movement toward a democratic agriculture is impossible without making both commodity prices and property transfers serve social goals. Thomas Jefferson desired that land be returned to a common pool for reselling after the death of the farmer. Not many societies have tried this solution, but many have taken farmland out of the market (that is, farmland could be passed on but not sold). In countries as different as China and large parts of rural Mexico, this is true today. In Sweden, local boards must approve farmland sales, ensuring that prices remain within the reach of farmers and that sales go to make more viable farms, not simply to enlarge the already profitable ones. Also in Sweden, only farmers can own farmland. In two of Asia's more successful economies, similar rules have made farmland no longer a mere commodity: In Taiwan and in South Korea, absentee ownership of farmland is not permitted. Sweden has also taken wholesale prices of agricultural commodities out of the market in order to provide the price stability on which family farming hinges. Commodity prices are determined when farmers' representatives sit down periodically with representatives from government, industry, and consumer cooperatives. Retail food prices, on the other hand, are set by the market except for certain essential foods like bread and milk, which are subsidized.

These brief examples illustrate a variety of approaches to the problem of injustices that the market system perpetrates on competitive producers when other sectors are highly concentrated, as well as injustices *within* agriculture that exist as long as farmland remains a speculative commodity. You'll notice that virtually all my examples are in countries that most Americans would call capitalist. Most have not done away with the market or with private property. What they *have* done is to reduce these absolutes of capitalism into flexible mechanisms, limited so as to protect democratic goals.[12]

These solutions to the problems of farming have positive ramifications for food consumers, too. Farmers freed from pressure to produce maximum volume in order to counter price fluctuations can concentrate more on the quality and wholesomeness of their crops. And, in a farm economy in which there is once again room for the family farmer, there is also room for more variety and diversity in what is grown and how it is marketed and sold. Consumers can thus enjoy what ought to be a wider range of more flavorful and more wholesome food. At the same time, restoring and protecting the local farm economy will allow us to revive local food sources and markets that have long disappeared under the tidal wave of supermarkets and chain restaurants, and to renew local and regional food traditions and flavors that can reawaken the pleasure and community once central to the table.

I firmly believe that so long as we define the problem of food and farming in narrow market terms—as, for example, simply increasing commodity prices, enhancing efficiency or convenience, or lowering consumer costs—we cannot envision a democratic system of food production and use in this society. Price itself is a misleading guide, and fairer prices themselves cannot address the property relations that determine the winners and losers resulting from a price increase. In fact, the vision that I am suggesting is not at base a set of market relationships at all. It is a set of ethical choices about what best serves our needs—what is fair to people and fair to the land.

Some will respond that you cannot talk to farmers about anything but the market and how to ensure that it brings them better prices. But my sense is that farmers are not unlike the rest of us. They know in their hearts that the current rules, built on a concept of an economic self with narrow economic interests, are not working. And those who have been around for a while know that farming is not just about economics. This is what many farmers are trying to tell us. If they had wanted to get rich, most would have chosen a different livelihood to begin with. The noneconomic values drew family farmers to their work in the first place and keep them there, sometimes against impossible odds.

Similarly, we are told that, for consumers, price, convenience, and appearance are everything. But everywhere there is evidence to the contrary. Survey after survey shows that Americans not only are concerned about the purity and wholesomeness of their food but also are willing to pay more than they do now to guarantee them. And the growing popularity of direct farmer-to-consumer marketing, witnessed by farmer's markets and roadside stands, shows that those same consumers are interested in where their food comes from and in the people who produce it. Increasingly, the connection between farmer and consumer *is* being restored, benefiting communities and the economy as well as being socially and aesthetically satisfying. Finally, at all levels of society—not just the wealthiest—people are interested in their food: in its provenance, its flavor, and its place in both their personal well-being and that of the community and the environment as a whole.

In spite of this, many continue to conclude that family farmers are quaint relics of the past. I conclude the opposite. In their protests, they articulate that what they are losing is what most Americans want, too: a way of life in which economic viability is only a vehicle, not an end in itself. The end is a life centered in family and community relationships and in responsible stewardship of that which ultimately belongs to none of us—the land itself. Clearly, consumers are expressing the same concerns and desires. In both cases, media, opinion leaders, and government seem not to have caught up yet with what is a flourishing, if often unarticulated, consensus.

My challenge is simply to ask you to be willing to consider that sustainable agriculture and a sustainable culture in which food — as it must be — is central are not just about terraces and hedgerows or supermarkets and recipes. But to do so, we must ultimately confront the most widely held assumptions about our very nature. Relying on our intuitive mistrust of those who would reduce human beings to their "economic selves," we can overcome our fear of taking on economic dogma. No longer intimidated, we can not only confront the injustices that a concentrated market economy brings down on competitive producers; we can also address how market relations themselves, used exclusively to assign value and define opportunity, undermine our vision of a democratic economy. As Thomas Jefferson argued, every generation is responsible anew for its governance. In facing this challenge to ourselves, I leave you with the words of philosopher Lewis Mumford:

> Our main handicap will be lack of imagination. . . . This is one of those times when only the dreamers will turn out to be practical men.

Notes

1. Susan Sechler and Ken Cook, "It's Time to Face the Facts: The Family Farm Is Doomed," *Washington Post National Weekly Edition* (Feb. 11, 1985), p. 23.

2. Personal communication to the author. Goodwyn wrote *The Populist Moment* (New York: Oxford University Press, 1978).

3. Statistics in this and the following paragraphs are from U.S. Department of Agriculture, "Economic Indicators of the Farm Sector," *National Financial Summary* (Washington, D.C.: Government Printing Office, 1984), pp. 13–14.

4. Marj Charlier, "More Young Farmers Rent Land They Till, Often to Avoid Debt," *Wall Street Journal* (Feb. 3, 1987).

5. Quoted in Roderick Nash, *The American Environment: Readings in the History of Conservation* (Reading, Mass.: Addison-Wesley, 1976), p. 51.

6. Food Marketing Institute, "Food Marketing Facts" (Washington, D.C., 1988).

7. Marshall Sahlins, *The Use and Abuse of Biology* (Ann Arbor: University of Michigan Press, 1976), p. 100.

8. Adam Smith, *Theory of Moral Sentiments* 1, (Edinburgh: Hay, 1813), p. 1.

9. Smith, *Theory of Moral Sentiments,* p. 194.

10. Charles Darwin, *The Descent of Man and Selection in Relation to Sex* (New York: Appleton, 1909), chap. 4.

11. This discussion benefits from the insights of environmental philosopher J. Baird Callicott, University of Wisconsin, Stevens Point. See, for example, *In Defense of the Land Ethic* (Albany, N.Y.: SUNY Press, 1989).

12. The preceding section benefits especially from the work of Marty Strange of the Center for Rural Affairs whose recent book is *Family Farming: A New Economic Vision* (Lincoln: University of Nebraska Press/Institute for Food and Development Policy, 1988).

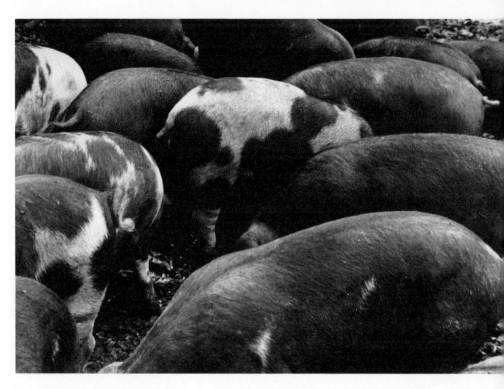

Pigs, Mechanicsburg, Ohio, June 1938. Photo by Ben Shahn.

A Resource Directory
Leslie Land

A Bibliography

Wendell Berry
The Unsettling of America: Culture and Agriculture
Sierra Club Books, 1977
The Gift of Good Land
North Point Press, 1981
Home Economics
North Point Press, 1987

Louis Bromfield
Malabar Farm
1948; reprint edition, Aeonian Press, 1976

Bruce Brown
Mountain in the Clouds: A Search for the Wild Salmon
Simon & Schuster, 1982

David Bulloch
The Wasted Ocean
Lyons and Burford, American Littoral Society, 1989

Rachel Carson
Silent Spring
Houghton Mifflin, 1962

Marion Clawson and Burnell Held
Federal Lands, Their Use and Management
1957; reprint edition, University of Nebraska Press, 1965

Jack Doyle
*Altered Harvest: Agriculture, Genetics, and the Fate of the
   World's Food Supply*
Viking Press, 1985

Denzel Ferguson and Nancy Ferguson
Sacred Cows at the Public Trough
Maverick, 1983

Terry Gipps
*Breaking the Pesticide Habit: Alternatives to Twelve
Hazardous Pesticides*
International Alliance for Sustainable Agriculture
(Minneapolis), 1987

Jim Hightower
Hard Tomatoes, Hard Times
Shenkman, 1972/1978

Robert West Howard
The Vanishing Land
Ballantine Books, 1985

Wes Jackson
New Roots for Agriculture
University of Nebraska Press, 1980
Altars of Unhewn Stone: Science and the Earth
North Point Press, 1987

Wes Jackson, Wendell Berry, and Bruce Coleman, editors
*Meeting the Expectations of the Land: Essays in Sustainable
Agriculture and Stewardship*
North Point Press, 1984

Mark Kramer
*Three Farms: Making Milk, Meat, and Money from the
American Soil*
Harvard University Press, 1980/1987

Frances Moore Lappé and Joseph Collins
Food First: Beyond the Myth of Scarcity
Ballantine Books, 1979

J. Tevere MacFayden
Gaining Ground: The Renewal of America's Small Farms
Holt, Rinehart & Winston, 1984

William McLarney
The Freshwater Aquaculture Book: A Guide to Small-Scale Fish Farming
Cloudburst Press, Hartley and Marks (Point Roberts, Wash.), 1984 (available through New Alchemy Institute—see "Appropriate Agriculture")

Laurie Mott and Karen Snyder
Pesticide Alert
Sierra Club Books, 1988

Gary Paul Nabhan
Enduring Seeds: Native American Agriculture and Wild Plant Conservation
North Point Press, 1989

Joe Paddock, Nancy Paddock, and Carol Bly
Soil and Survival
Sierra Club Books, 1986

Marc Reisner
Cadillac Desert: The American West and Its Disappearing Water
Viking Press, 1986

R. Neil Sampson
Farmland or Wasteland: A Time to Choose
Rodale Press, 1981

Orville Schell
Modern Meat
Random House, 1985

Marty Strange
Family Farming: A New Economic Vision
University of Nebraska Press/Institute for Food and Development Policy, 1988

David Weir and Mark Schapiro
Circle of Poison: Pesticides and People in a Hungry World
Institute for Food and Development Policy (San Francisco), 1981

Organizations and Periodicals

General

Here it pays to heed the injunction: "Think globally, act locally."
Regional resources are often the strongest, both for general in-
formation about what's going on and for specific help in finding
suppliers, growing your own, and so on. Stellar examples are the
Northwest's **Tilth** (4649 Sunnyside N., Seattle, WA 98103, [206]
633-0451) and the **Natural Organic Farmers Associations**—of
New York and all the New England states (information through
NOFA–NY, P.O. Box 454, Ithaca, NY 14851, [607] 648-5557).
These and similar groups in the South, Midwest, and elsewhere
are listed in:

Healthy Harvest No. 3 is a considerably larger version of the
first two editions of this small guide. Over a thousand listings in
forty-one categories, from small seed companies and individual
organic farms through resource libraries and research bodies to
global organizations such as Oxfam. Entries from more than
thirty countries and all fifty states. Potomac Valley Press, 1424
16th St. N.W., Suite 105, Washington, DC 20036. $18.95
postpaid.

The following sections offer slightly more specific resources
(by topic).

Appropriate Agriculture

Institute for Alternative Agriculture: Focused on research and
education, publishers of a scholarly quarterly and a very handy,
mercifully brief monthly newsletter full of tidbits about current
legislative activities, academic goings-on, and so on. Quarterly,
$20; newsletter, $15; both, $30. 9200 Edmondston Rd., Suite
117, Greenbelt, MD 20770, (301) 441-8777.

Land Institute: Research and education center founded by Wes
and Dana Jackson, addresses a broad spectrum of ecological and
agricultural issues but is especially focused on perennial grain
crops and an understanding of and respect for the prairie. Newsletter, *The Land Report,* three times per year for $6. Annual,

The Land Institute Research Report, describes and analyzes the year's experiments, $2.75. 2440 E. Water Well Rd., Salina, KS 67401, (913) 823-5376.

New Alchemy Institute: Famous for its interest in integrated systems for producing food, shelter, energy, and the like in sustainable ways. Primarily educational. Membership ($35) includes quarterly newsletter, reduced tuition for courses, and discount on publications and products. 237 Hatchville Rd., East Falmouth, MA 02536, (617) 564-6301.

Rodale Press/Regenerative Agriculture Association: This mixed (profit/nonprofit) complex of publications, research institute, and consultants is probably the largest, best-known, and longest-running citizens' advocate of appropriate agriculture in America. *Organic Gardening,* the original magazine ($14.97/yr.), is now glossier, more sophisticated, and less dogmatic about what's natural and what isn't. *New Farm* ($15/yr.) addresses commercial farmers' concerns from an earth-cherishing perspective that is also fully respectful of the bottom line. Both magazines include many news bites of interest even to those who neither garden nor farm. 33 E. Minor St., Emmaus, PA 18049, (215) 967-5171.

Biological Resource Preservation

American Minor Breeds Conservancy: Works to preserve and increase stocks of uncommon farm livestock. Publishes *Minor Breeds Notebook* ($8) with information on four-footed types, *Poultry Census and Sourcebook* ($4) about the winged branch. Bimonthly newsletter with membership, $20. Box 477, Pittsboro, NC 27312, (919) 542-5704.

Environmental Policy Institute: Works on a broad range of agriculture and water-quality issues, mentioned here because of its efforts to have us look carefully at biotechnology before leaping into the brave new world of engineered crops and livestock. Base membership ($10) brings monthly newsletter. 218 D St. S.E., Washington, DC 20003, (202) 544-2600.

Native Seeds/SEARCH: Focused on conservation of crops and farming practices of native populations in the Southwest. Membership, including quarterly newsletter, $10; seed catalog, $1. 2509 N. Campbell Ave., Suite 325, Tucson, AZ 85719, (602) 327-9123.

North American Fruit Explorers: Membership organization mostly involved with research and cultivation, though preservation of old, rare, and noncommercial varieties also gets some attention. Initial one-year membership ($11) brings you a handbook and the quarterly *Pomona,* which contains research reports, queries, and so on from active-grower members. Route 1, Box 94, Chapin, IL 62628; 10 South 055 Madison St., Hinsdale, IL 60521, (217) 245-7589.

Seed Savers Exchange: Grassroots organization devoted to saving heirloom seeds. Members ($15/yr.) exchange material through annual yearbook, get two other publications, have access to plant-finder services. Publishes mammoth *Garden Seed Inventory* ($17.50/paper) and *Fruit, Berry, and Nut Inventory* ($19/paper). Route 3, Box 239, Decorah, IA 52101, (319) 382-5990.

Farmland and Farm Culture Preservation

American Farmland Trust: Conserves farmland through public policy initiatives, information aid to activists, and outright purchase or covenanted resale of prime farmland. Membership ($15) includes quarterly newsletter. 1920 N St. N.W., Suite 400, Washington, DC 20036, (202) 659-5170.

Center for Rural Affairs: Focused on public policy. Sponsors publications and projects devoted to small-farm preservation. Monthly newsletter (suggested donation, $20) covers all aspects of small-farm policy including foreign trade. Quarterly ($10) features in-depth analysis of farm finance issues. P.O. Box 405, Walthill, NE 68067, (402) 846-5428.

Rural Advancement Fund: Devoted to small-farm survival, genetic resources preservation, and related public policy.

Quarterly newsletter, free. 101 East Salisbury St., Pittsboro, NC 27312, (919) 542-5292.

International

Greenpeace: Included because of its efforts to stop pesticide misuse in less-developed countries. 1436 U St. N.W., Washington, DC 20009, (202) 462-1177.

Institute for Food and Development Policy/Food First: 145 Ninth St., San Francisco, CA 94103, (415) 864-8555.

R.A.F. International Communiqué: Monthly publication of Rural Advancement Fund (see previous section), covering socioeconomic impacts of biotechnology in the third world. Subscription, $20.

Worldwatch Institute: 1776 Massachusetts Ave. N.W., Washington, DC 20036, (202) 452-1999.

Meat and Fish

Alternative Aquaculture Association: Membership ($12/yr.) brings a quarterly newsletter. P.O. Box 109, Breinigsville, PA 18031, (215) 395-5854.

Defenders of Wildlife: Listed because of their interest in preserving American rangelands from the devastation wrought by poor grazing practices. Membership ($20) includes bimonthly magazine. 1244 19th St. N.W., Washington, DC 20036, (202) 659-9510.

Food-Animal Concerns Trust: Helps livestock producers with humane growing, avoids moralizing, stresses economic benefits of alternative animal husbandry. Wholesale-markets (but not for profit) appropriately raised veal and eggs; will refer callers to retail sources of their own or others' products. P.O. Box 14599, Chicago, IL 60614, (312) 525-4952.

National Fisherman: The industry magazine and biased accordingly, but full of useful hard news about landings, legislation, and the latest in technology. (Not nonprofit.) Thirteen issues/year, $19.95. Editorial offices, P.O. Box 908, Rockland, ME 04841-0908, (207) 236-4342.

National Sea Grant College Program: See listing under "Water Quality and Preservation."

Pesticides

Americans for Safe Food: Part of the Center for Science in the Public Interest. "Safe" as in contaminant-, pesticide-, and drug-free. Primarily a lobbying organization, with secondary emphasis on consumer education. Publishes guides to mail-order sources of organic produce and naturally-raised meat ($.50 each, plus business-size SASE with $.50 postage) and booklet ($5), *Organic Agriculture: What the States Are Doing,* which provides brief overviews of action at the state level along with a list of useful contacts. 1501 16th St. N.W., Washington, DC 20036, (202) 332-9110.

National Coalition Against the Misuse of Pesticides: Primary focus on consumer education. Newsletter five times a year with $20 membership. 530 7th St. S.E., Washington, DC 20003, (202) 543-5450.

National Pesticide Telecommunications Network: Twenty-four-hour help line with information on all aspects of pesticides, including health and environmental effects. Their answers tend to be specific in direct relation to the specificity of one's questions. Partially funded by the Environmental Protection Agency but not committed to the party line. Free booklet, *Citizen's Guide to Pesticides.* (800) 858-7378.

Water Quality and Preservation

American Rivers, Inc.: Dam fighters primarily, but concerned with fisheries and water-quality issues as well. Quarterly newsletter, $20/yr. 801 Pennsylvania Ave. S.E., Suite 303, Washington, DC 20003, (202) 547-6900.

Clean Water Action Project: Community and lobbying organization. Quarterly newsletter, $24/yr. 317 Pennsylvania Ave. S.E., Washington, DC 20003, (202) 547-1196.

National Sea Grant College Program: There's one in almost every state that has a coastline, including those on the Great Lakes. All sorts of original research, data collection, and publications. For information on the nearest, contact the director's office: 6010 Executive Blvd., Room 812, Rockville, MD 20852, (301) 443-8925.

Other Organizations
Given the deadly effects of agricultural pesticides on birds, no one should be surprised that the **Audubon Society** is an active advocate of appropriate farming. **The Natural Resources Defense Council** not only concerns itself with the likes of Alar but also publishes the *Farm Land Preservation Directory* for the Northeastern United States. Similarly, other organizations from the **Sierra Club** to the **League of Women Voters** all devote some of their resources to encouraging appropriate food production.

Contributors

EDWARD BEHR (*A Sense of Place*) is a writer on food and other subjects and is editor of the widely praised newsletter *The Art of Eating*.

WENDELL BERRY (*The Pleasures of Eating*), one of America's foremost spokesmen on sustainable agriculture, is a poet, novelist, and essayist whose books include *The Unsettling of America, A Place on Earth, The Gift of Good Land, Standing by Words, Remembering,* and, most recently, *What Are People For?*

BRUCE BROWN (*The Last Columbia Salmon*) is a Pacific Northwest–based journalist and the author of *Mountain in the Clouds: A Search for the Wild Salmon*. His book on the American farm crisis, *Lone Tree: A True Story of Murder in America's Heartland,* appeared in fall of 1989.

ROBERT CLARK (*Editor*) is editor of *The Journal of Gastronomy*. A former medievalist and newsletter publisher, he is currently working on a biography of the late James Beard, to be published by Harper & Row.

GRETEL EHRLICH (*Growing Lean, Clean Beef*) is the author of *Heart Mountain,* a novel, and *The Solace of Open Spaces,* essays. She has been published in *Harper's, Atlantic,* the *New York Times,* and *Time.* She and her husband, Press Stephens, ranch in northern Wyoming and have been involved in holistic resource management for three years.

PAUL GRUCHOW (*Remember the Flowers*), a writer and journalist based in Worthington, Minnesota, is the author of *A Prairie Year* and, most recently, *The Necessity of Empty Places*. A frequent public speaker on agriculture and wilderness, he has regularly been featured on National Public Radio.

WES JACKSON (*Making Sustainable Agriculture Work*), co-director of the Land Institute in Salina, Kansas, is the author of *Altars of Unhewn Stone: Science and the Earth* and *New Roots for Agriculture* as well as the editor of *Man and the Environment* and, with Wendell Berry and Bruce Coleman, *Meeting the Expectations of the Land: Essays in Sustainable Agriculture and Stewardship*. One of the leading figures in the movement for sustainable agriculture, he holds graduate degrees in botany from the University of Kansas and in genetics from North Carolina State University.

MARK KRAMER (*Are Farmers an Endangered Species?*), author of *Three Farms: Making Milk, Meat, and Money from the American Soil* and of *Invasive Procedures: A Year in the Life of Two Surgeons,* is writer-in-residence at Smith College.

LESLIE LAND (*A Resource Directory*) is a nationally syndicated newspaper columnist and the author of *Reading Between the Recipes*. She writes frequently on food, gardening, and the environment for the *New York Times, Metropolitan Home,* and other national publications.

FRANCES MOORE LAPPÉ (*Food, Farming, and Democracy*) is the author of the bestsellers *Diet for a Small Planet* and (with Joseph Collins) *Food First: Beyond the Myth of Scarcity*. She heads the Institute for Food and Development Policy/Food First in San Francisco. Her most recent book is *Rediscovering America's Values*.

ANNE MENDELSON (*Paradise Lost: The Decline of the Apple and the American Agrarian Ideal*) has been a frequent contributor to *The Journal of Gastronomy* and to other publications on food and related topics. A food historian, she is currently working on a biography of Irma S. Rombauer and Marion Rombauer Becker, the authors of *Joy of Cooking*.

GARY PAUL NABHAN (*Food, Health, and Native-American Agriculture*) is the assistant director of the Desert Botanical Garden in Phoenix and a cofounder of Native Seeds/SEARCH. He won the John Burroughs medal for natural history in 1985 for his book *Gathering the Desert*. He is also the author of *The Desert Smells Like Rain: A Naturalist in Papago Indian Country* and, most recently, of *Enduring Seeds: Native American Agriculture and Wild Plant Conservation.*

ALICE WATERS (*The Farm–Restaurant Connection*) is the founder and guiding force behind Chez Panisse in Berkeley, California, one of the nation's most influential restaurants, and has consistently focused attention on the dependence of all cooks on first-rate materials. She is the author of *The Chez Panisse Menu Cookbook; Chez Panisse Pasta, Pizza, and Calzone;* and, with Paul Bertolli, *Chez Panisse Cooking.*

WILL WEAVER (*The Gleaners*) is the winner of prizes from the McKnight and Bush foundations, the National Endowment for the Arts, and the PEN Fiction Project. He is the author of a novel, *Red Earth, White Earth,* and a collection of stories, *A Gravestone Made of Wheat.* He lives in Bemidji, Minnesota.

Acknowledgments

All of the following essays appeared in *The Journal of Gastronomy,* Volume 5, No. 2 (Summer/Autumn 1989):

"A Sense of Place," copyright © 1989 by Edward Behr. Reprinted by permission.

"The Pleasures of Eating," from *What Are People For?* by Wendell Berry, published by North Point Press. Copyright © 1990 by Wendell Berry. Reprinted by permission.

"The Last Columbia Salmon," copyright © 1989 by Bruce Brown. Reprinted by permission.

"Growing Lean, Clean Beef," copyright © 1989 by Gretel Ehrlich. Reprinted by permission.

"Remember the Flowers" was first published as "An Excellent Life" in *Minnesota Monthly.* Copyright © 1989 by Paul Gruchow. Reprinted by permission.

"Making Sustainable Agriculture Work," copyright © 1989 by Wes Jackson. Reprinted by permission.

"Are Farmers an Endangered Species?" copyright © 1989 by Mark Kramer. Reprinted by permission.

"A Resource Directory," copyright © 1989 by Leslie Land. Reprinted by permission.

"Food, Farming, and Democracy," copyright © 1989 by Frances Moore Lappé. Reprinted by permission.

DATE DUE

APR 15 2			
GAYLORD			PRINTED IN U.S.A.